THE
HEALTHSHARING
READER

D1785710

THE HEALTHSHARING READER

Women speak about health

Compiled by
Healthsharing Women
Publishing and Production Group

PANDORA

SYDNEY   WELLINGTON   LONDON

To all those women who have worked for the health
of women in Australia.

First published in Australia by Pandora Press, an imprint of the
trade division of Unwin Hyman Limited, in 1990.

Copyright © Healthsharing Women 1990

All rights reserved. No part of this publication may be reproduced,
stored in a retrieval system, or transmitted in any form or by any
means, electronic, mechanical, photocopying or otherwise, without
the prior permission of Unwin Hyman Limited.

Condition of sale: this book is sold subject to the condition that it
shall not, by way of trade or otherwise, be lent, re-sold, hired out or
otherwise circulated without the Publishers' prior consent in any
form of binding or cover other than that in which it is published, and
without a similar condition including this condition being imposed
on the publisher.

Allen and Unwin Australia Pty Ltd
8 Napier Street, North Sydney, NSW 2059, Australia

Pandora Press
Unwin Hyman Limited
15–17 Broadwick Street, London W1V 1FP, England

Allen and Unwin New Zealand Limited
75 Ghunzee Street, Wellington, New Zealand

National Library of Australia
Cataloguing-in-Publication entry:

Healthsharing reader: women speak about health.

  Includes index.
  ISBN 0 04 442154 0.
  1 Women—Health and hygiene. I. Healthsharing
  Women
613.0424

Set in 10/11.5 Plantin by Midland Typesetters, Maryborough
Victoria
Printed by Dah Hua Printing Press Co. Ltd, Hong Kong

Contents

Foreword

Germaine Greer

Twenty years ago I wrote a book called *The Female Eunuch*. Its argument, which most people misunderstood, was that women as we know them are castrated; their energy, or libido, or life force, or *élan vital*, being irrelevant to their domestic function, has been destroyed or diverted into unproductive channels by a long and ineluctable process of conditioning. This argument has to presuppose a female genotype (woman as she could be) which is realised only in a distorted form in the phenotype (woman as she is). My book, and my feminism, are continuing acts of faith in the existence of an unknown creature, the whole woman. Twenty years have not brought us to the emergence of the whole woman from oppression, repression and mutilation; not for nothing has the women's struggle been called by Juliet Mitchell the longest revolution. Nevertheless we can congratulate ourselves. The process of liberation has begun and some important ground has been taken and held. *The Healthsharing Reader* is evidence of the progress that has been made.

First of all, *The Healthsharing Reader* is evidence of women's growing awareness that they are more than daughters, girlfriends, wives and mothers; they are first of all women, who feel first of all solidarity with other women, no matter what their orientation or role in life. Women ought not to be a minority group, because they are not a minority, but as long as they are subdivided, into categories related to the services that they render to the patriarchal family, they amount to no more than a series of overpopulated minority groups and are manipulated accordingly. *The Healthsharing Reader* is evidence of a concerted attempt to break down the barriers erected between women and women, the barriers of race, class and culture, as well as of marital status, sexual orientation and age.

Next, and almost as important, *The Healthsharing Reader* has striven to be a co-operative effort. The evidence of experts is here given the same weight as the evidence of uneducated women, some of whom will be seeing their thoughts on paper, let alone between the covers of a book, for the first time. The key is 'learning from each other', health workers learning from patients, patients learning about health workers, women learning from women.

The aim of health-sharing is to allow women finally after centuries of enforced childishness to take responsibility for their own health and the quality of the contribution they make to life on the planet. It may never be possible to say that women have control over their bodies, for bodies do not always behave in predictable or controllable ways, but women will one day be able to say that their bodies are not in the control of anyone else, that no foetus has the right to invade them, that no man has the right to penetrate them, or to use them for fun or profit, that no one can imprison them, that no one can poison them with chemicals or insert gadgets in them without the woman herself desiring it, not merely giving consent more or less informed, but desiring it.

The corollaries of taking responsibility for one's wellbeing are many and fundamental. Wellbeing entails happiness, or rather, given the world's load of guilt and grief, serenity. Care of the body is inseparable from care of mind and soul. Perhaps it is not too soon to look forward to a day when women's mental suffering will not be dealt with symptomatically by the administering of tranquillisers, as more and more women come to realise that doctors cannot prescribe antidotes to injustice.

Health is a political question, not simply because the provision of health care is directly or indirectly the business of governments, but because the pressure of political structures bears directly upon the individual citizen's mind and body. Patriarchal oppression is manifest at every phase of the female citizen's development, from the time she opens her eyes upon our world. Her attitude to her own developing faculties, her strength, her intelligence, her independence, is shaped from the outset by the situation into which she is born.

The Healthsharing Reader adopts the most rigorous feminist criteria as part of a necessary strategy to exorcise self-blame, the most insidious result of female conditioning, and therefore makes possible, if at a still very distant remove, the emergence of a proud, strong, self-regulating female human, who will be at one with her body, who will give her own account of the menstrual cycle, be sexually active when and how she wants, give birth when and how she wishes or not at all, and approach the great climacterics of menopause and death without anxiety or induced helplessness, using the enormous resources of modern medicine to encompass her own aims rather than to serve someone else's convenience and priorities.

Acknowledgements

Project Co-ordinator: Linda Martin. *Project Committee:* Maria Bohan, Freya Headlam, Helen Myles, Rose Sorger, Kathy Wilson. *Interviews:* Maria Bohan, Linda Martin, Panayiota Romios, Rose Sorger, Kathy Wilson. *Editing:* Christine Gillespie, Freya Headlam, Linda Martin, Helen Myles, Kathy Wilson. *Illustrations:* Seren Trump, Deborah Kelly, Judith Rodriguez. *Photography:* Joyce Agee. *Graphics Co-ordination:* Freya Headlam, Rose Sorger. *Compilers:* Teresa Capetola, Clare Carberry, Suzanne Cooper, Tricia Szirom. Thanks to Gretchen Guest, Margaret Howell and Bonnie Simons.

Contributors

IRENE BOLGER, a union activist, was secretary of the Victorian Branch of the Australian Federation of Nurses from 1986 to May 1989. She has been a charge nurse in several hospitals and taught at the Alfred Hospital School of Nursing.

MARJ THORPE is active in the Aboriginal Rights Movement. She is currently employed as a research assistant in mental health by the Aboriginal Health Service in Melbourne.

OLGA KANITSAKI, a nurse, was born in Crete. She migrated to Australia in 1961. Olga is a lecturer in the Department of Nursing, Lincoln School of Health Sciences, La Trobe University.

CORAL BENNETT taught primary school and, with her family, ran the general store in Wandiligong, Victoria until 1974. She co-authored *Wandiligong, A Valley Through Time*. Coral was awarded the Medal of the Order of Australia in 1989 for her work in conservation and welfare.

DESLEY PAANASAE lives in Papua New Guinea and works with the East Sepik Women's Network.

ROMA CUSACK (pseudonym) trained as a teacher. She is currently a senior book editor with an educational publishing firm. Prior to that she was co-ordinator of a community newspaper.

JUDITH JONES works at the Social Biology Resources Centre in Melbourne. Her current focus is on education about the prevention and management of AIDS and other sexually transmitted diseases.

SUE WRIGHT is a senior lecturer in health education at Melbourne University. She was formerly a research officer with the Royal Australian College of Obstetricians and Gynaecologists and a curriculum development officer in health education for the Victorian Ministry of Education.

HELEN MYLES is a nurse with extensive experience in health education and equal opportunity. As a member of the Clarity Collective she is co-author of *Taught Not Caught* and *Feeling Good About Yourself*.

DEBORAH DAVISON is in work-related child care and has been involved in youth work and sexuality education. She is a member of the Clarity Collective and co-authored *Taught Not Caught* and *Feeling Good About Yourself*.

FIONA STRAHAN is the executive officer of the lobby group STAR, Victorian Action on Intellectual Disability. She is involved in political issues concerning women, disability and social justice.

JUDITH RODRIGUEZ lectures in English and Australian literature at the Royal Melbourne Institute of Technology and also teaches creative writing. She has published seven books of poetry. Her latest anthology, *New and Selected Poems*, was released by the University of Queensland Press in 1988.

LISA CHEN (pseudonym) is a community worker. She is interested in Chinese culture and medicine. She lives with her partner and three children.

MARY MAHONEY is a community educator with Action for World Development. She is involved in the peace movement and a women's consciousness-raising group.

SUE EVANS and ASSUNTA HUNTER are herbalists with degrees in social sciences. Both lecture at the Southern School of Natural Therapies in Melbourne.

PATRICIA CROTTY is a lecturer in nutrition at Deakin University. She has worked as a dietitian in hospitals, community health centres and the Health Department of Victoria.

ROSLYN BAYLISS is a general practitioner in rural Victoria. A native of Coffs Harbour, Roslyn graduated from the University of New South Wales in Sydney.

MARGARET GODING trained as a clinical psychologist. She works as a feminist therapist in a community health centre in Melbourne and has a small private practice. She has two young children and is a member of the Feminist Therapy Collective and Family Therapy Group in Melbourne.

LINSEY HOWIE is an occupational therapist and a Gestalt therapist. She lectures in occupational therapy at the Lincoln School of Health Sciences, La Trobe University. Linsey is a member of the Feminist Therapy Collective and has three teenage children.

GAI MAYES lives in rural Victoria where she is involved in writing and music.

LORRAINE GREAVES is a sociologist teaching and writing in London, Canada. She is active in the international women's health network. Lorraine is the author of *Background Paper on Women and Tobacco*.

BEATRICE FAUST was a founder of the Women's Electoral Lobby and was president of the Abortion Law Repeal Association. She is the author of *Women, Sex and Pornography*.

GWENDA HIGGINS is the director and co-founder of TRANX (Tranquilliser Recovery and New Existence) Inc. of Victoria, which was established in 1986. Gwenda has a background in nursing and drug and alcohol rehabilitation.

DIANE GRAHAM (pseudonym) was a teacher and has recently trained as a health worker.

KATE GILMORE is co-ordinator of the Centre Against Sexual Assault (CASA House) in Melbourne. As a community worker, she is active in women's health issues in both a paid and unpaid capacity.

SHAMIMA ALI is a founder of the Women's Crisis Centre in Fiji, which opened on 13 August 1984.

SANDY GIFFORD is a lecturer in the Department of Social and Preventive Medicine at Monash University. She has conducted research in the areas of screening for breast and cervical cancer.

JAN SOUTHGATE is a social worker. She researched a discussion paper called *The Teaching of Medical Students to Conduct Pelvic*

Examinations for the Victorian Health Department. Jan is currently co-ordinator of the Outer Eastern Women's Health Service in Melbourne.

JO WAINER is the executive director of the Abortion Providers' Association. She works with the Fertility Control Clinic in Melbourne.

THE PENINSULA HOMEBIRTH SUPPORT GROUP OF FRANKSTON, VICTORIA was founded in June 1988 by Jenny Fawkes. It is a non-profit organisation with approximately twenty members.

RENATE KLEIN is a research fellow in women's studies at Deakin University. Her most recent book is *Infertility: Women Speak Out About Their Experiences of Reproductive Medicine.*

ROBYN ROWLAND is a senior lecturer in women's studies at Deakin University. Her latest book is *Woman Herself, A Transdisciplinary Perspective on Women's Identity.*

All interviews were conducted by the staff of Healthsharing Women.

Introduction

Over the past months, a group of us has worked to draw this book together. The resulting anthology interweaves strands of political analysis with personal voice and theory with experience. It acknowledges the truth and importance of women's lives and the effect of health on women's daily living.

The women who wrote the articles, and those who talked together, each added to the definition of women's health; as their views and experiences flooded in, our task of selection became huge.

The pieces finally selected were chosen both for their individual impact and their complementarity. The book is divided into sections and the articles in each section are linked by theme or topic. Connections also occur from section to section and this connectedness reflects women's ways of knowing and learning. Some pieces can be read quickly and absorbed, whilst others require more concentration. Like pieces of a jigsaw, when fitted together, they create a larger picture of women's health.

Women's health issues are woven into the social, political and economic environment. Much of the ill-health—emotional and physical—suffered by women is generated by the world around us: infertility is viewed as a crisis, abortion as a moral issue judged by the state, and questions related to contraception are decided on the basis of 'acceptable' population levels.

In choosing the contents of this book, we have tried to illustrate that while on one hand women's health involves increasing rates of breast, cervical and lung cancer, idiosyncracies of the reproductive system, sexual transmission of disease, diet or depression, on the other hand certain issues underpin women's health and ill-health.

Discussion of the relationship between 'healers' and women occurs frequently, and consequently the issue of control over women's bodies arises again and again. The role of medical science, and of medical practitioners within that science, is often questioned, and strong messages for health professionals emerge from the voices of ordinary women in this book.

Many of the pieces highlight the power of information or the lack of it, and plant the seed that 'facts' as they are told to us are in reality values of the dominant culture, parading as 'truth'. It is possible to trace the process by which women's knowledge and control over their health has been usurped by men and machines. This current climate of control is evident in a number of sections which capture industrial, violent, reproductive and psychic dimensions of women's health.

Yet this book is not about defeat or women as victims. If, as women, we had relinquished control over our bodies and our lives, then these stories would not have been told. Many of them are tributes to the courage and persistence of women, and the book as a whole celebrates women's understanding and action.

We acknowledge that we have not covered in depth or breadth all the issues involved in women's health or represented the diverse range of women's experience. For each piece included we received several others, and our thanks go to all the women who offered their contributions. This book is for them and women everywhere.

Part I

Taking Action

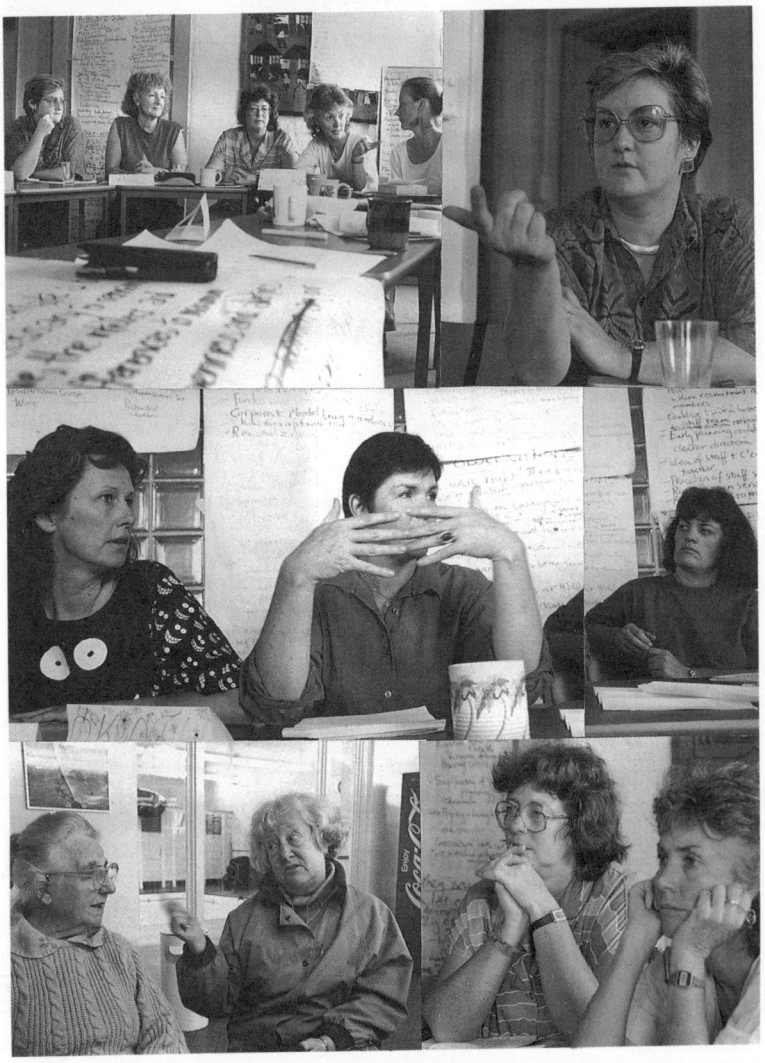

Women, Joyce Agee, 1989

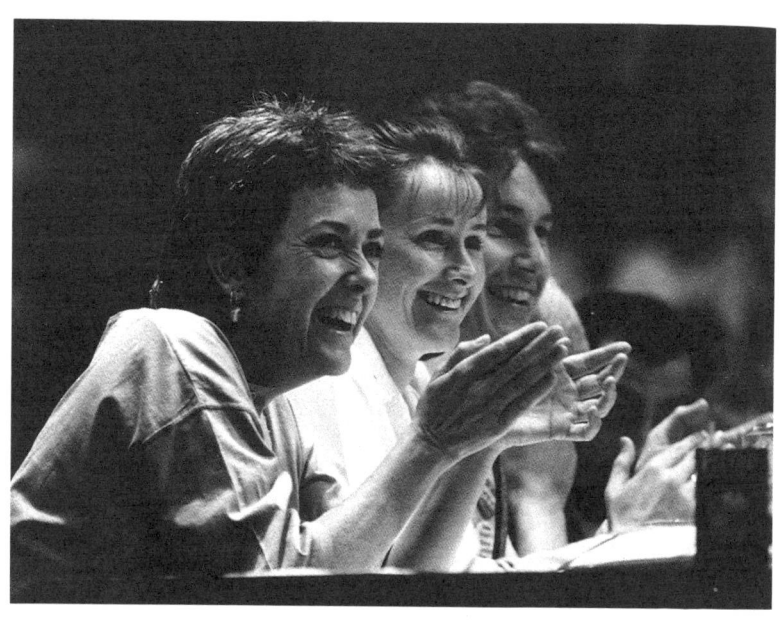

Above: Irene Bolger (left) and colleagues

Below: Victorian nurses on strike, 1986

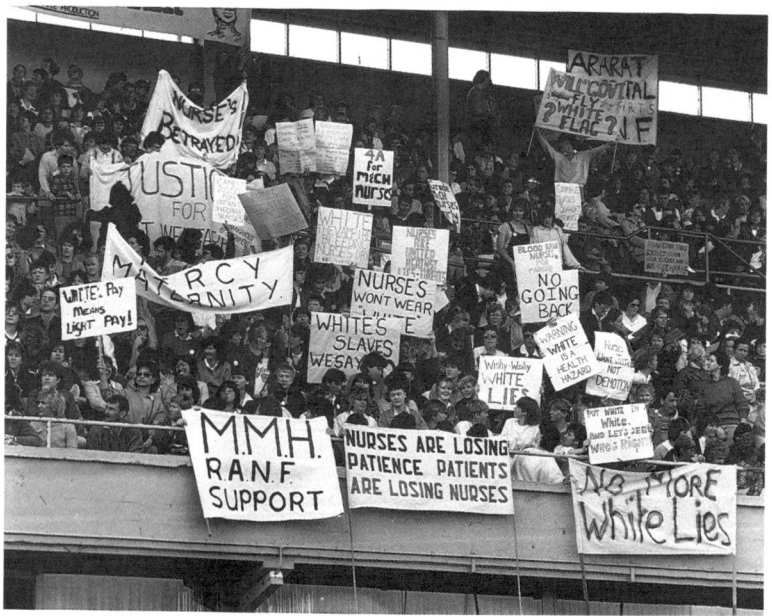

Nurses strike!

Irene Bolger interviewed by Rose Sorger and Linda Martin

In October 1986, Irene Bolger, secretary of the Victorian Branch of the Royal Australian Nursing Federation (RANF), called Victorian nurses out on strike. Four months earlier, there had been an arbitration decision to downgrade nursing positions. This affected nursing awards and caused pay inequalities between major hospitals and all other hospitals. Allowances for midwifery and other special care were reduced. There were to be no pay increases for students or recently qualified nurses.

The nurses were immediately pressured to return to work. They were threatened with the Essential Services Act. David White, then Minister for Health, appeared on television and demanded that the RANF negotiate. Personal attacks against Irene Bolger were frequent and vicious.

On 15 December 1986 the Australian Council of Trade Unions (ACTU) and the Nursing Federation submitted a joint proposal to the government. Behind-the-scenes negotiations were moving favourably for the nurses and, on 19 December, the members voted to return to work.

On 23 January 1987 the Industrial Relations Commission accepted the major part of the ACTU and Nursing Federation's proposal. Previously demoted nurses were upgraded under a new career structure. Student and recently qualified nurses were to have reasonable pay increases. Special care allowances were restored. Nurses would move to professional pay rates over the next two years, and the government and the RANF commenced a study into professional nursing which was completed in February 1988.

Linda: Irene, you came under a massive personal attack as the leader of the nurses' strike. Why do you think that happened?

I think the hostility was a combination of things. I know that it was partly political, because we were breaking out of the Accord.

That was seen as a political threat by the state government and also by the ACTU, because the ACTU wanted to keep the lid on it, as they still do.

My being a woman was also a focus for attack. They tried to make it look as if I didn't know what I was doing, and that nobody in their right mind would challenge the system. Because I was a woman I was supposedly terribly naive about the real industrial world and the danger in taking the nurses down this 'path of destruction', which included bringing down the Accord.

An incredible amount of male hostility was directed at me. David White had a lot of difficulty actually looking straight at me and speaking to me. So a tactic he used was to look at some man, perhaps a male industrial officer with me. He would speak to this man and I would have to say, 'Listen, you're talking to me, look at me.'

He found me incredibly aggressive and at times I was; you had to be, otherwise you would be squashed. They would say you were weak if you didn't stand up to them. But when you did stand up to them, they would call you unfeminine. They found me so difficult to deal with because I wouldn't buckle under. The media also has this really peculiar idea about the way women in industrial relations are supposed to behave. So there was the full spectrum of media treatment, from ridiculous articles about who was in love with me to equally ridiculous articles about whether I was able to cope. Did I cry? Was I stressed? These were questions they would never ask a man. The media followed me around all the time. Journalists became fascinated with this idea of a woman running a strike of that magnitude and I don't think they ever did come to terms with it.

Linda: Did you have personal support through the strike?

There was a circle of friends and there were also members of the union who used to be really very supportive. My son was fifteen at the time. I'm a single parent. There were the day-to-day problems of housework. I was spending up to eighteen hours a day in and out of the Arbitration Commission, on picket lines and negotiating. So there were these people who were incredibly supportive behind the scenes, making sure my son was fed and the house was cleaned.

Rose: In the initial stages of the strike the nurses decided not to wear their uniforms. I heard there were a lot of sexist comments by some of the doctors and administrators such as: 'Well, at least it's a change and we get to see women's bodies.'

Yes, it was amazing. The reaction generated was fascinating. They hated nurses being in civilian clothes. The male paternal attitude was that they must be in uniform so that everybody could place them where they really belonged in the system.

Rose: Has there been a backlash against nurses who went on strike?

These nurses don't get on to committees. They miss out on jobs all the time. The pressure was on them from the day they walked back into those hospitals after the strike. They had to contend with going back in just before Christmas to find that the scabs who had been working then had made a fair bit of money and were able to take Christmas off, go away, and have a holiday.

A heavy guilt trip was laid on them about walking out and leaving patients. There was always a core staff, not to mention the doctors on duty, so no lives were in danger.

Rose: Were people surprised to see how politically committed nurses were to the strike?

Absolutely. There was a gross miscalculation on the part of the Health Department, the government generally, Left politicians as well as Right politicians, other unions, the public, the media. Everybody grossly underestimated the determination of the nurses. The fact that I was elected should have been warning enough. Still, nobody believed the members would follow me out. They thought that since we were females and nurses we would be wimpy.

But I understood where these nurses were coming from and the conditions they had been dealing with. I'd been a nurse myself for about twenty years. When I was running for election and talking to nurses, I had a good sense of their mood. I saw it was time for action because they'd had enough. I knew there was a lot of anger, and nurses were ready for change. That's why I was elected and that's why nurses walked out of the hospitals.

Rose: Yes, that walking out was very strong when it was seen on the television: nurses flooding out of the hospitals. It had a dramatic and symbolic quality that was extremely powerful.

It was partly industrial instinct and partly knowing how to use the media. We knew which hospitals were prepared to go out. We'd choose one at random so the Health Department didn't get on to it, then do a press release. Everyone else would collect in the front foyer at the beginnng of the shift. Then the staff would walk out and we'd clap and cheer and support them. A lot of them were crying. We thought, we're going to show you, en masse, this is what it means to us. It was so difficult for nurses to do it. Yes, the symbolic walk out was very potent.

3

Linda: Was the nurses' strike symbolic for women in general?

There's no doubt. I've been invited to speak about the strike interstate as well as in Victoria. The strike is seen as being significant in terms of women's place within the industrial relations system. There hadn't been recognition that women were an integral part of the union movement, but suddenly the men had to sit up and take notice. Other unions contributed to our strike fund. I think the strike gave heart to a lot of other union women. It made them feel it's worth struggling on and that they can do something.

I'm on the Trades Hall executive and often I've been the only woman there. The men have had to accept me but even the Left frequently takes an opposing view to mine. I've found that I'm often the odd one out. When it's time to vote, everyone else has their hand up except me. So I've developed a thick skin.

They find it difficult to accept that women really do have a meaningful part to play, that women do have an understanding, and can participate. At least the men listen more now. They have to.

Women burn out really quickly in the union movement because they don't have the same network as the men. There's a lot of good women around. It's just a matter of trying to keep in contact or we tend to get isolated. Anyway, the nurses' strike gave a lot of women a lot of heart.

Rose: What was the political climate like during the strike?

There wasn't much sympathy, even from the Left. I was hauled in front of the Left parliamentarians' caucus three times to be told that there wasn't enough money to give in to the nurses' demands.

Linda: So you were getting pressure from the media, from the government, from the Left. What about police harassment?

The police harassment was interesting because I think it was also political. At the beginning of the strike, Cairns was the one who was put in charge of our strike. He contacted me very early on and asked us to co-operate to a certain extent. I finally told him to shove it after the nurses were bashed on the picket line at the Royal Melbourne. Usually it was the local police who patrolled the picket lines. They were friendly and chatty with the nurses. But two days before our mass meeting the special operations group of the police appeared at the Royal Melbourne. They kicked and punched, pulled hair, and dragged women around—nasty stuff. This got an enormous amount of publicity on the news. It was done to frighten the nurses so they would give in.

Rose: How did the general public react to the strike?

The strike put a lot of strain on the public's goodwill towards nurses. There was also some abuse. I used to get death threats every day. Some of them were taken more seriously than others. There were probably about five serious ones. There were times when I had to have my car or house searched because of a bomb threat. One day I was at the Commission and wondered why the police suddenly appeared. Apparently somebody had said they were going to shoot me there. There was a death threat against my son. That really got to me. I was so nervous. I used to get in my car in the morning and hesitate. I'd have to steel myself before turning the key in the ignition. My car could have blown up. I used to get men ringing up saying, 'Get married. If you got married, you'd be satisfied and stop all this nonsense.' My whole life changed so dramatically to the extent that I was total public property. I had no privacy at all. But I was so single-minded about the strike that I could cope with all that stuff.

Linda: Did the strike raise the consciousness of nurses?

Yes, not of every nurse of course, but a significant number. Since the strike, politically within the RANF there's been a very strong move away from industrial action. There is a group of nurses, particularly in management, who want to pull back. They often say that the public view of us is that we are not caring enough anymore. They talk about professionalism. But they won't be more assertive, or fight for control over what happens to nurses in hospitals. For example, nurses should be on hospital ethics committees and participate in decision-making at every level.

This faction wants to be less confrontational and more accommodating. Some of them have trouble accepting a woman as a boss, as a leader. So there's more conservatism, resulting in attempts to remove me.

Rose: What have been some of the tactics used in trying to get you out?

I was accused of financial mismanagement. There was this consistent leaking of selected information to the media, and they ran with it. It began in 1988 with a series of articles in the *Australian* about funds' abuse. This is why I would never resign. Because the information was false.

John Jost ran two programs, in the style of an exposé of Irene Bolger and the RANF. The line of questioning that Jost took made it seem like the strike fund had been misused. This wasn't true, but the members were asking, 'What's going on?' So it was bad publicity.

Nothing has ever been proved against me. I've consistently said that if their allegations were true, they could have sacked me. They could have charged me. Of course, they haven't because there were no real charges.

There are personal attacks as well. People don't talk to me. A lot of rumours are spread around about my personal life, like who I'm supposed to be having an affair with. The pressure is incredible— very hard to deal with. By the end of 1988 I wasn't coping at all. I had to go into hospital to try and sort myself out. But I still keep on. It drives my opponents insane because they thought I would resign.

Linda: What sustains you?

I believe in what I'm doing. My motives are positive. I have tried to do what I think is right. I'm up for election in October 1989 and I'm going to run again. It will be a fairly hot election. There have already been rumours around that somebody's been offered money to get photos of me with this particular man. The focus on my sexuality started with the strike and has continued. Right from the beginning the media seemed fascinated by whom I might be sleeping with.

Rose: It seems there is also the notion that women can't manage money, that they don't have those sort of administrative skills and that women don't have staying power. You know, women eventually give in or get broken.

That's right. But what is never recognised is that when I was elected, the RANF was twenty years behind the times in lots of things. We didn't even have our membership records computerised. When I came in I was faced with a very inefficient organisation, as well as being confronted immediately with the longest strike in our history. We had to buy staff cars and a computer. We had to spend money on upgrading the Federation. And we had a very expensive strike so that cost us money too. The Federation is in debt but so are many unions after a strike.

Within the RANF the male influence is becoming more predominant. About 5 per cent of nurses are male. In the hospital system it's disturbing, because they move through the system much quicker than women. About 99 per cent of them will have senior managerial positions within a couple of years of their graduating.

Rose: Do you think it's a special gravitational force?

Yes, hot air rises! What's interesting is, since we've made significant gains in wages, there have been more men coming into nursing.

Linda: Can you discuss what some of the conditions for nurses are like now?

There's a very high turnover. It's got a lot to do with things like lack of proper child care, and the stress of the workloads. More women are dropping out of the full-time workforce and taking up part-time work. This is a real problem because the more part-time workers you have, the less industrially strong you are. These workers only want to go and work their couple of days, get their money and go home.

Linda: What about doctor–nurse relationships?

There's some sexual harassment. For instance, I remember in an operating theatre a doctor squirted a syringe full of water up a nurse's dress. That's not an isolated incident. I've experienced harassment too. You might be going on a ward round, and you'll get a pat on the bum. Now if you say, 'Get your hand off my arse' they think you're overreacting. Doctors wouldn't like it if you stuck a hand up between their legs. But when they fondle nurses they think it's funny. And it's not just touching. It's sexist jokes as well.

Sometimes surgeons scream at nurses in the operating theatre, throw instruments at them, and take all their stress and aggravation out on the nurse. They can be incredibly rude and dictatorial. It happens in every hospital.

The part that I found very difficult about being a nurse was that my opinion was never valued. That doctors thought that if you were a nurse you were too dumb to be anything else. I think that one of the things that came out of the strike is that doctors have a bit more respect for nurses. There are still an awful lot of doctors out there who are against nurses upgrading their education or nurses having any decision-making power. But that's slowly changing.

Linda: Do you think women who would have been nurses in the past are now going into medicine and becoming doctors?

No, you might even find it's the other way round. I know a woman who was a doctor and then switched to nursing, saying it was more satisfying work. There's been an overintellectualisation of medicine. Emotionally, nursing can be a lot more rewarding because of the close contact with patients. I think that some more sensitive, enlightened doctors see that. Many doctors have become personally removed from their patients and there has recently been an attempt in medical education to address this.

It isn't easy even for nurses to focus on a patient's needs and comforts. The routine of the hospital still takes precedence over the needs of patients. As a patient, you're dependent on nurses for everything, so you don't want to offend them. There's a long way to go, but I think there is more recognition of patient's rights.

Rose: Well, what is the way ahead for nurses?

I think the concept of power and how to use it has to be picked up by nurses. We have to get over the post-strike guilt and build on what we learned.

Postscript

A few months after this interview, on 24 May 1989, Irene Bolger was sacked as state secretary of the Australian Nursing Federation. The ANF union's state council found Bolger guilty of several charges of breaching union rules. Bolger intends to fight the sacking in the Federal Court and she has appealed to the rank and file of the union to support her.

A matter of survival
Koorie health

Marj Thorpe interviewed by Maria Bohan

Marj, how did you become active in Koorie issues?

In the 1930s my grandmother and later my mother were both involved in the Aboriginal rights movement. My brothers and sisters and I had a good teacher in our mother. She was always behind us and always encouraging others as well.

We lived in the country during my childhood but we had contact with our extended family in Melbourne and throughout Gippsland. We grew up with the feeling of Aboriginal community.

When I was a teenager I became involved with the Aboriginal Advancement League. During school holidays I got a job as a receptionist with the League. I was only about fifteen and the late 1960s were exciting years because a lot was happening in the area of Aboriginal issues. Later I worked in the Aboriginal Legal Service when it first opened.

Around 1976 I moved on to the Aboriginal Health Service. We started up a clinic in the 1970s for child and maternal health. We encouraged women, mainly at home with very young children, to get out, meet and talk about their problems or interests. At the same time their children would have checkups, have their growth recorded, and be immunised. Out of that, the child-care course has developed.

Why was there a need for a specific health service for Koories?

They weren't getting proper access to the existing services. We were finding that children weren't getting adequate screening and mothers weren't attending antenatal clinics. A lot of mothers hadn't had any checkups or visited any doctors during their pregnancies.

Much of that stemmed from the attitudes of white professionals within health institutions. It was the way they treated Koories, from outright racism to paternalism. Obviously people are not going to seek medical treatment when they're feeling intimidated in any way.

Aboriginal women would still have their babies mostly in hospitals, wouldn't they?

Yes. And even now the attitudes of the nursing staff and some doctors are terrible. Of course that doesn't apply only to Koorie women. I've seen a lot of other women being victimised because they can't speak English, for example. I think the health professions have a lot to answer for.

There should be clinics set up in the Aboriginal Health Service and other community health services so that those women can receive the care that they deserve and feel comfortable with.

If you were going to set up those clinics, attached to Aboriginal Health Services, what would you need?

You would need the personnel, the equipment and money. You need to have adequate funding to provide those things. Women are going to hospitals because there's no other choice. And there are a lot of women I know who refuse to go to hospital unless it's an emergency. They come to the Aboriginal Health Service instead. But that means we are confronted with situations that should be hospital cases. Women even want to have their babies at the Service or at home, rather than go to hospital.

How do Koories feel about using their own Health Service rather than mainstream systems?

Before our service was set up, someone would go to a doctor and talk about lots of other things without coming to the real reason why they were there. People comment that it's much easier to relate to the doctors we have, obviously because they have some under-standing of Koories. They've been hired for that reason. People are much more able to be at ease and tell the doctors what is really wrong with them.

There's a social atmosphere at the Aboriginal Health Service. It's not only a medical situation. People who go there can talk with others and not feel so isolated.

Non-Koorie Australians have a lot to learn from what Koories have fought for and discovered in relation to health.

I think there's been some instances where they've taken blueprints of what we have developed, especially in community health care. And some non-Aboriginal people are even using our service, particularly from the Housing Commission flats.

What are some of the other health issues specific to Koorie women?

There is a high tendency for Koorie women to suffer from diseases like diabetes, high blood pressure, alcohol and drug addiction and psychological problems. These come from the socio-economic situation that we are in, including the white society's denial of our culture, dispossession of our land, lack of educational and employment opportunities, and the horrifying history of genocide that we can't forget.

There is also a concern about sexually transmitted diseases. Because we are a small close-knit community, diseases like AIDS are a real threat to us. If something like that gets into our community, the effects are going to be devastating. There's a special unit within the Health Service to deal with this. We are educating the Koorie community about AIDS and trying to prevent it from spreading.

Working in the area of Koorie health must be quite demanding.

I think that the people who work in community-controlled organisations have that real commitment. There's no way they're going to toss their jobs in here. It gets really hard and frustrating but we support each other. Our own health suffers and that affects our families. But there's no way these people will turn their backs on our cause and work where it's easier or the money's better. You've still got the old die-hards who never give up. And that in itself makes you feel you're not the only one. There have been times when there just hasn't been money for salaries, cleaning, rent—basic things like that. It's terrible. The government lets us down sometimes and they play mind games. And you can always see through it.

Do Koorie women meet separately from men sometimes—to talk about health issues for instance?

Not really, no. That's been one of the things we don't want to buy into. We need to be united. Some women's groups and resources were established. And where that has been attempted, it's caused a lot of problems because the men feel threatened. So if men want to be involved they're not knocked back.

There's an initiative at the moment to build a new child-care centre in Thornbury. Can you tell me anything about that?

My sister is the co-ordinator of the Yappera Day Care Centre. It's a small place in Fitzroy. There's really only space for sixteen children. Well, there's always more than that there. The parents of these kids are working so the kids have to be there.

The centre is right in the middle of factories in a really dirty area. So there's talk of developing a new complex in Thornbury. It would include a day care centre, a kindergarten and a pre-school. Women have been saying that they want a specific clinic for themselves that they can go to and talk about their own health problems. This could be part of the complex.

It would be a community-controlled facility. If you don't have the people themselves initiating the programs and implementing them, then you really don't have anything much different from what we've already got. We've proved with the organisation of the Health Service that people with no education whatsoever are able to achieve what government and medical administrators couldn't do.

They tried to provide adequate health care for Aboriginal people before. It didn't work. Aboriginal people had a go at doing it and they proved to be successful under enormous pressures such as inadequate wages. You don't even get funded for the most critical types of services you might need. I mean real basic stuff like cleaning or enough money to pay the rent.

We spend a lot of time dealing with the bureaucracy, and that takes away from the time we need for the service. It's one of the biggest problems that's faced. I can't understand the thinking in that, because what we've also proved is that we're providing a much cheaper standard of care on a dollar-for-dollar basis.

Marj, what developments are you looking forward to in Koorie health care?

There is a shortage of Koorie health-care professionals. So now we have a training program at Koorie Kollij. This will help provide health care to people who have no access to any care whatsoever. These skilled people go back to their communities and at least you've got somebody who knows when medical treatment is necessary. Too often kids and adults got sick and died because no one knew what to do.

What keeps you going so that you can continue on with the struggle?

It's part of my life, and my children's lives. The whole family is involved. I've got no choice. You can't walk away from it. My job isn't nine to five. I can't leave it behind when I go home. Most people who work in this organisation don't do it for the money, because there's certainly not much of that. It's a matter of survival. We've got to work for change.

Dignifying difference
Multicultural health care

Olga Kanitsaki interviewed by Panayiota Romios

Can we begin by talking about your life experience and how that has affected your understanding and contributed to your knowledge about ethnic women's experience of health care in Australia?

Well, when I came here to Australia in 1961, I was seventeen and I was full of dreams and knew very little about Australia. There were films in Greece before we immigrated—all these beautiful, huge landscapes with horses running around, the richness of Australia, Sydney Harbour, the nice streets, ice creams, nicely dressed kids and women. It was just beautiful propaganda to attract immigrants, it's as simple as that.

So the reality was different from your expectations?

It was nothing like I imagined. When I came here it was an incredible feeling, as if I was an alien in another world. Isolation, loneliness, no meaning, I couldn't communicate because people wouldn't understand—almost like being on the moon. There was little support, only a few relations, a few friends. I didn't know how to get a tram from my corner to go into the city. I remember in the beginning I was unemployed for six months. Once I learnt how to, I caught the 6.30 tram every day to the city to look for a job.

Eventually a girl I knew who worked in Cooleys' Pies got me in there. I was there for six months cleaning onions by hand. And I had always been very healthy, I never had headaches or sore throats. But once I went there I started to get these terrible headaches and my eyes were very red. I didn't realise it was the onions. They wouldn't move me. I used to leave work with the most terrible migraines, vomiting. I'd tell them, 'I'm going home.' I'd be sick for a day or two, take a pill, then get up and go to work again.

The irony was that in order to immigrate you had to be perfectly healthy. They were very strict about that because they wanted strong workers. But the work itself made us feel ill.

Also, I used to work irregular hours. We didn't know our rights. We thought that if we said anything, they'd kick us out and then we'd have nowhere to go, to eat, to sleep. And because we knew nobody and nothing about the system, our fears were enormous. You can't imagine it. We were so frightened, we would work under any conditions and we wouldn't complain.

In Greece you ate when you were hungry and slept when you felt tired. I wasn't used to having such a rigid structure. It was a strange concept for me that there were specific times for lunch or for morning or afternoon tea.

So I left there. I was unemployed for another three months. Then I went to another factory called Holeproof where I used to tie knots all day. I remember going to the toilet and the boss would say, 'Hurry up, hurry up'. He'd come and knock on the toilet door. You had to get up very quickly and you didn't have time to wipe yourself. I know now, because I'm a nurse, that quite often, because of hurrying, a lot of women got urinary tract infections. If you wear jeans or tights, and you don't wipe yourself properly, it's an ideal medium for the growth of micro-organisms. A lot of women actually were scared to take one minute extra.

It's still a big issue. It hasn't changed. I've heard women talk about it.

Exactly. They don't know the system or realise that they have rights like any other human being. Sometimes people will say things have changed now. But what has actually happened is that the workers have adapted.

Anyway, when I was in the factory, women used to get terrible headaches because of the unbearable noise. If you wanted to talk to someone, you had to shout at the top of your voice.

Quite often, they used to pick out an immigrant and make them a boss, a leading hand. And because they were as scared as everybody else, they were worse than the other supervisors, driving the workers saying, 'Hurry up, don't do that, don't say that, because they'll kick you out.' So the women were even more afraid.

Even worse was the sexual harassment on that job. One day the boss actually told me that he wanted to see me nude in the bath. This was 1964. A friend of mine in the factory said she was forced to sleep with him in order to keep her job. I was so scared when I heard this, that I resigned. I went to work as a machinist where my sister was working. I asked to sit next to an Australian woman to learn English. They sacked me from there because I was talking to this woman and they didn't want you to talk.

After that, I went to the Children's Hospital through another girl-friend. I started cleaning the lockers. My friend and I lived in the same room and shared the same bed. We couldn't afford anything else.

I worked in the Children's Hospital for about two years. That's when I realised that I could study. 'How can I become a nurse?' I asked. I approached the matron, and she said that I didn't speak sufficient English to go into nursing. So I started to learn more English at that time from another Greek person I knew.

I really wanted to be a nurse, so I went to Fairfield Hospital and spoke to Vivian Bullwinkle. She gave me the opportunity to start my nursing aide's course—that's the state enrolled nurse now.

I still couldn't speak much English. In class the first day, the only words I understood were Greek terms in anatomy and physiology. The other students were all Australian. I was working all day, and then I would study till three o'clock in the morning to translate word by word, using a dictionary, the lessons I had learned from English into Greek so as to be able to understand them.

I had to lock myself in the toilet, because it was lights out at eleven at night. One night the night supervisor caught me and I had to see Miss Bullwinkle the next day. I thought I was going to be kicked out. But that woman—I will never forget her. She asked me why I was in the toilet, and I told her. So she said, 'OK, you promise me you will study only until two in the morning and I'll let you have the light on.' She wanted to be sure I got some sleep so I wouldn't get sick, seeing that I had to start work at 7.00 a.m. She had suffered during the war. She understood what I wanted to do, and she gave me a chance. By the end of the year I was the top of the class, I got a distinction.

Then Miss Bullwinkle encouraged me to do more nursing, infectious diseases, and I got a distinction again. I spent three years before I went on to general nursing, studying English and Australian culture, so I could communicate with people and get the right messages across. I spoke a bit more English by then, but I still had a lot to learn. A woman said to me one day, 'I'm only pulling your leg', and I said, 'No, you aren't, you're not even touching me!' Understanding English is to do with a shared culture, a shared history.

Then I went to PANCH [Preston and Northcote Community Hospital] and did my three years' training as a nurse. At that time I worked with a lot of immigrant patients. I understood them so deeply, my heart was crying for them, my soul was going out to them when I saw them, particularly the old people. In Greece, I knew another culture, and that made me sensitive about the needs of other people whose cultures I didn't know.

What were your working conditions like?

There was a lot of prejudice. They used to say to me, 'Speak English', when I tried to help an elderly woman or man who couldn't speak English, by translating into Greek. The staff thought I was talking about them.

I realised that there were reasons why people I worked with behaved the way they did. In order to understand their insecurities I had to ask how I could help them, rather than becoming defensive or angry about their behaviour.

I remember from about 1970–1974 I was working in casualty, and we had two Greek doctors there. I knew they spoke Greek, but they were too scared to. It was that bad. People looked at you oddly if you spoke another language. One time, this Greek doctor went to see an old Greek man, and he was speaking to him in English. So I went up to him and said in Greek, 'Aren't you ashamed to speak to him in English when he doesn't understand? I'm disgusted with you.' I was a registered nurse then and I knew a bit more. They knew my stance in the hospital.

Because they didn't have translators, I was doing two jobs. They take advantage of you and you know it. But you still do it willingly, even though you tire yourself out. You work a double shift. I was there as a registered nurse, not as an interpreter. But how could I not go, when I knew what these people were going through?

And even now they are using hospital cleaners to translate. They don't realise that interpreting takes skill and training.

Also, understanding people is more than just a matter of language isn't it?

Yes. It reminds me of a story about an Italian woman who couldn't eat her lunch. I knew for us Greeks that bread was a basic food item, especially for elderly people. My mother couldn't eat a meal unless she had bread. So I realised that this woman needed a piece of bread with her meal. I went to the nursing sister, and asked her to ring the kitchen for some bread. The woman ate her meal, but the sister complained, saying, 'Why can't this woman eat her food like all the other patients?' The problem is, we interpret equality as treating each person the same as everybody else. That's wrong, because that is exactly how inequalities can arise.

When people won't recognise cultural differences, cultural needs?

Yes. For equality, you must recognise the differences and then do whatever you can to provide for those different needs. If a person's culture is not respected, they slowly lose their identity, their self-esteem, their self-image, because so many of their experiences are negative.

For example, a lot of immigrants start getting headaches, backaches and muscular pains because they do long periods of repetitious work. When I was working tying knots, I began to get a lump on my bone. When I stopped, it stopped growing. It was caused by my job, but I didn't know that or that you could take them to court or do anything about it. I was just a young girl.

It still happens with immigrants working. They start getting pains in their muscles, and until recently doctors haven't believed them—some still don't. They send them to psychiatrists or psychologists, or give them tranquillisers, or other drugs. The woman goes home and says 'He didn't believe me. He thinks I'm crazy.' It's a vicious circle.

Is it only language and cultural differences that create this situation?

I don't believe that's all. Doctors and other health professionals or helpers often see the world from one point of view—the way they were trained. They are not prepared to accept diversity, or to see cultural differences. They feel that what they offer is superior, and anything else that the patient may want or may know is inferior. That is ethnocentricism. I'm not saying all health professionals are like this, but there are some.

How do we make changes?

We need people who know about cultural differences and are prepared to do something to get laws passed. I am the president and founder of the Transcultural Health Care Council, an organisation which started in 1985. We are a group of about 55 health professionals who saw all these problems and thought, 'How can we change things? Let's unite and see whether we can do something about it.' It's open to everyone and we would like to have patients too, so they can express their values and opinions, so we can fight for change together.

What we have to do now is to educate the community, to raise the issues and make both sides aware—health professionals and immigrants.

What is on your agenda?

We have to tackle the issues at government level—policy changes, law reform and institutional changes. For example, we need informed consent forms in other languages so patients can understand them. What happens now is they say to them 'Put a cross here.' So they sign it without knowing what they are signing for. We need menus in hospitals in different languages so people can at least choose what to eat. Just very simple things like that.

Also, in many cultures, collective decision-making by the whole family is a traditional support for the individual. To deny a patient this support would be like asking an Australian to cut off an arm or a leg before they went to hospital. A person may want to discuss whether or not to have an operation with their entire family so they can all decide. The law of informed consent in Australia expects everyone to behave like a sole individual. This needs to change.

But laws don't affect attitudes do they?

You need to change the law, but you also need change in institutional procedures reflecting attitudes. For example, a rule might say only two visitors per hour. That's based on the idea of the individualistic nuclear family in Australia. If you go to a Greek hospital, they have no limits on visitors. Policy makers in hospitals need to look at these rules and draw up changes.

Has there been any response from the government to the Council's submissions?

We drew up a basic framework for nursing education and policy initiatives in public health institutions, including items such as re-cruiting qualified nurses from overseas, from different ethnic back-grounds and with two languages.

Last year the Health Department of Victoria commissioned two large enquiries. One was regarding the medical profession and the other, the nursing profession. In the nursing enquiry, nothing was included from our submission. I was very upset about that so I rang the minister. We have been involved in interdepartmental discussions and now we are writing a new refined framework to submit.

We must sensitise the people who are in power and who can do something. We should go to the conferences and give papers. Last year I gave a variety of papers to staff and students at public hospitals and universities. Slowly you get the message through. But it's not enough. We really need commitment to affirmative action and struc-tural changes.

I'm fighting hard to include cultural anthropology, cultural attitudes, into the curriculum. They tell me that I can have six hours. They forget that they have sociology for 120 hours, 250 hours for psychology. But whose sociology, whose psychology? The Anglo-Australian, not the immigrant. There needs to be a multicultural approach across the curriculum which would eventually be reflected in practice.

Can you outline a transcultural health care model?

The model would be an acceptance of diversity with holistic care by a a wide range of different health-care workers. A lot of folk medicine is psychologically and socially beneficial. We cannot ignore these remedies, because once we say that we don't accept them, really we are saying, 'We don't accept you.'

Once I saw a Vietnamese woman who had taken her child to the hospital. He had a high fever, and the doctors didn't know what was causing it and they couldn't lower his temperature. The mother kept asking for a Vietnamese healer to be called in. The doctors didn't want to, but finally one agreed. The boy's temperature came down. The doctors were amazed. They kept him in the hospital for a few more days to see if it was just a coincidence, but he stayed well and finally he could go home.

Would a woman of non-English speaking background be more disadvantaged than other people in the community in relation to health?

There is no doubt about that. She is disadvantaged in terms of her class because of poverty and lack of information about available services. It's a matter of degree. I go to the hospital. I have an accent, I'm a woman and I'm uneducated. I find certain disadvantages because of my accent, because I'm a woman, and I'm in a powerless position. But I'm white. If I was a woman, had an accent, and was black, lesbian or elderly, I would be worse off.

Race, gender, age—all of these make up a person's culture which determines their values and identity. The closer you are to the dominant, white, male culture, the better you understand how to operate within that system.

We need to change our mainstream systems to fulfil the needs of people of various cultures and thus there is a need for transcultural health-care workers. It's not that their needs are so different—everybody gets hungry, everybody has pain—but their needs are satisfied in different ways. That has to be accepted.

Breathing free
The fight against pesticides

Coral Bennett

The signs of the coming rat race were clear to us when 42 years ago my husband and I and our small daughter took a big step and left the city and our teaching jobs. We were opting for life in the country as proprietors of a general store in Wandiligong. This tiny hamlet in north-east Victoria has been our home ever since and here our family of five children grew up. Life was quiet and peaceful until the radio report on 25 July 1981.

It was a lazy Saturday morning and we decided to stay in bed until after the local news from 2CO. We were stunned to hear the announcement that aerial spraying of 2,4,5–T was about to take place

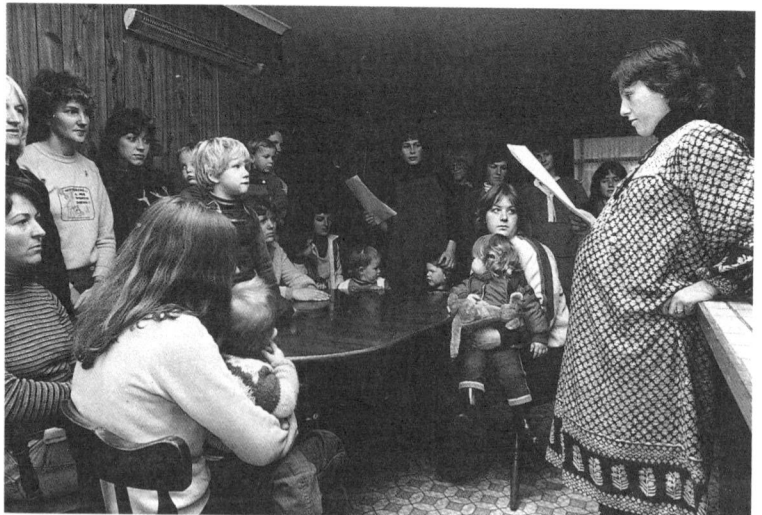

Residents meeting comprising of Bright and Wandiligong mothers and their children discussing the spraying, 1981. Photo from the *Border Morning Mail* by Rob Elliott.

over pine plantations in our district. This toxic herbicide is one of the components of Agent Orange, a chemical weapon used by the United States during the Vietnam War. It is suspected of causing birth defects and cancer.

I dressed hurriedly, muttering all the while 'Oh no,' and planning what should be done. I first checked with the radio station to see if we had heard correctly. There was no mistake. An informant had rung the station to report that he had been approached by a member of the Forestry Commission (now part of the Department of Conservation, Forests and Lands) two days before for permission to use his farm paddock as a helicopter pad for the spraying of plantations. Knowing something of the possible dangers of 2,4,5-T spray, the landowner refused this request.

A weekend is not the best time to get information, but most people know someone who knows someone else who works somewhere, and so by that evening we knew the specific area of the proposed spraying. The aim was to eradicate wattle suckers which were growing in the pine plantations. Pine plantations or softwoods have been part of the district since 1917, when unemployed men who had been gold mining planted out tracts of dredged and degraded Crown land.

The news of the proposed spraying spread rapidly throughout the district. The Wandiligong Preservation Society took on the job of organising the protest and asked for support. An ad hoc committee fell into place as the nursing mothers, playgroups, housewives, school parents' clubs and many others offered to help. The participants in the campaign were mainly women,well aware that they and their children would be the ones most at risk from the effects of chemical spraying.

On Monday the situation became clearer and we began to see what we were up against. The *Aerial Spraying Act* prohibits aerial spraying of certain herbicides after 31 July each year because of possible adverse effects on agriculture after that date. In this area that meant tobacco crops. We were incensed to learn that people rated less than tobacco. We later heard that a handful of families living on the edge of the plantation had been informed and that two had chosen to 'go away' during the spraying. The possible effect on the rest of us was not considered to be important.

Telegrams to MPs and the Forestry Commission were despatched and a strategy worked out. All the while we watched the skies, hoping the wet weather would continue to keep the waiting helicopter grounded until the allowed time ran out for spraying. The committee divided into groups as different women accepted responsibility for various tasks. The media coverage increased hourly and was handled by two people.

Scientific, professional and legal people from all over Victoria supplied us with information and advice. A district solicitor offered to act on behalf of the group and on Tuesday a written request was sent to the Forestry Commission asking that the spraying be called off pending a proper investigation into the possible effects of the spraying program. As we waited for a reply, our campaign grew in numbers and in volume. The reply arrived Wednesday afternoon, 29 July: spraying would go ahead.

The tension increased as we waited for either rain or the helicopter. But all the while we were organising and gathering support. The reply from the Forestry Commission left us with only one way to go: to seek an interim injunction order from the Supreme Court in Melbourne. A Wandiligong expectant mother agreed to take the main role in court and preparations were made to leave at daylight on Thursday. Signatures were being collected for what amounted to a blank cheque to pay court costs estimated to be anything up to $3000 at that time.

We were all upset and apprehensive but also determined. Someone suggested, 'You must get on to the Premier.' He was out of town for a few days, so I kept trying other contacts, pointing out that media coverage was already intense with plenty of negative publicity against a government department.

At 7 p.m. on Wednesday our solicitor got the message that the spraying for 1981 would be called off. Nobody really asked how the decision came about. Success!

Despite the victory, a public meeting already planned and advertised was held in the Wandiligong Hall on Saturday 1 August. The hall was crowded and there was a lot said. Husbands showed support for their wives and the action they had taken. This was not a minor thing, as many amongst the campaigners and in the audience owed their livelihood to the Forestry Commission. Some of the statements and claims made by the top bureaucrats and experts were false. They must have underestimated the knowledge and abilities of those in the audience.

Perhaps one of the most moving moments of the meeting was when a woman read Article 12 from the Universal Declaration of Human Rights (1948). This deals with the rights of people against arbitrary interference with family and home.

What was the fallout after the campaign? The pub talk became personal as family members were told that I 'needed my head read' and that other local women who had taken a lead in the campaign were 'ratbags'. Some families were divided over the issue as many forestry industry workers were involved. The discussion widened as soldiers who were victims of the Agent Orange disaster during the

Vietnam War related their tragic experiences. Letters continued to pour in from all over Victoria giving personal observations of the effects of 2,4,5-T.

In May 1982, the newly elected government curtailed the use of all aerial spraying of 2,4,5-T and its use in misting machines, and reduced the level of dioxin contained in the spray. Dioxin is highly toxic and causes birth defects. The government also tightened up sales controls.

A new range of sprays is being used today, namely Lontrel and Velpar. We have been told that they are safe, but many believe that it is the same old tale. So the fight against herbicides must continue.

The families of the Ross River and Stanley could write a sequel to this story, of their dramatic bid to prevent aerial spraying of pine plantations in November 1988. Seven years after the Wandiligong campaign, the use of herbicides is one of the major concerns facing country women and their families.

People often say that they feel powerless, especially in the face of government, big or small. However, the fact is that a very tiny place like Wandiligong could be the pivot for a campaign which pulled in active support from so many people. The campaigners, predominantly district women, generated enough energy to bring about important legislative change, showing that size has nothing to do with power. Each woman does have the power to do something about issues which affect her life.

Learning from each other

Desley Paanasae interviewed by Maria Bohan

Desley, can you tell me first, something about your background?

I was born in a north-east province of the island of Papua New Guinea (PNG). We left our village in 1966 and settled in Medina which is near the middle of the island. My father was working as a carpenter and my mother was a cook for the high school. They were just casual labourers. I was a student.

Were you able to do further studies?

I went to a girls high school in Port Moresby [the largest city in Papua New Guinea]. Then I went on to college to do my Diploma in Social Development.

Did you have to pay for your education?

Yes, as far as Year 11. When I went to college I had a government grant.

Would many people in Papua New Guinea have the opportunity to go on to tertiary education?

No, I think it's a lack of colleges. Even a lack of high schools. It's a very big problem.

Desley, you've recently been living and working in the East Sepik region of PNG. Would you describe what it's like there?

East Sepik is in north-west PNG. A river goes through the area and it's near the sea. The people are famous for the carving they do. The people who live on the coast have different features from those who live along the river.

What are the people involved in day to day?

Most people are farmers. All they do is work in their gardens, look after the children, look for food—everyday things. The men go hunting. The women do all the fishing, cooking and getting water.

Are there any industries in the region?

No, there are not very big companies around, compared to the other provinces.

Desley, what are some of the struggles or difficulties that people in the East Sepik region have?

One difficulty is no roads. So it's hard to get medicines or health care. Another problem for village people is communication. Most people don't own radios and don't hear about what is going on in other parts of PNG.

On the other hand, videos and television are coming in. I don't think many of the programs, especially the violent ones, are a good influence. I think there are enough problems, and we don't need to get any more ideas. They make our young people think that what they see on videos is real life.

In East Sepik, do most young people go to school?

There is no school. Eighty per cent of our people in Papua New Guinea cannot read and write and 80 per cent live in rural areas. Most women can't read. In our culture, if it comes to choosing whether a boy or a girl goes to school, it's usually the boy. That's because women are supposed to get married and look after the children. Most girls in East Sepik are not allowed to go away to school even for a few years because there is the fear that they might get into trouble.

What do women talk about when they are meeting with their friends?

They talk about food and where to go fishing. They complain about what the men are doing. They gossip a little bit, talk about their children or their worries. But they don't feel confident about gathering together in large groups. It's usually just a few women talking at one time.

What do men usually talk about?

I'm not very sure, because in our culture women are not allowed to hear what men say. The women cannot go very near.

If men and women are together socially or at a meeting, who does most of the talking?

The women do the listening, the men do the talking.

Desley, tell me something about the East Sepik Women's Network program that you have been involved in.

The network started in 1973 with three women. None was educated. They were having this problem with the government authorities who wanted the whole land to be planted with nothing but rubber. But these women knew food had to be planted too.

They visited each other and said, 'What can we do?' When they walked around to their neighbours, they found that a lot of other people were also worried. They said, 'OK, let's get together and share this.'

This network now consists of ten women who are leaders and five other women like me who work along with them. We have another five men who support us in our work, usually the husbands of these ten women. We emphasise helping each other.

A nutrition program was started. The group also learned to save energy by using charcoal instead of firewood for cooking. The people here live at a subsistence level and our program is bringing improvements.

Are women learning from and teaching each other?

Yes, and it has given them confidence. We started involving women from other districts who were interested in the program. They went back to their villages and started running workshops.

What has happened to the women who've been involved in the program? Have there been any changes for them?

Oh, yes. One lady and her kids had a skin disease. She learned about eating a balanced diet in the nutrition program and tried it on her family. They don't have skin trouble anymore. I wouldn't say everyone's health has improved but there are some changes.

Change takes a long time. Have the men felt left out of the program?

In some ways, yes. We try as much as we can to make the men happy. It's just part of our culture. But we have to make sure that they don't take over.

Have you had any difficulty with some men feeling very threatened?

At the provincial level, in the government especially, the men are so frightened. I think it's because we now have women who have never had any formal education, who are able to co-ordinate programs in the village. And these programs are becoming popular and successful. They feel that women are gaining status in the population and it's a threat to their own power.

Once a man broke into the building where I work and held a knife to my throat. He was so angry about the women's program.

You are very courageous to face that hostility. Is the East Sepik type of program happening in other parts of PNG?

There are a lot of programs in Papua New Guinea but the difference is that our program was started by rural women and then spread to the town. Other programs start from the town areas and then decentralise. And usually they are run by women who are married to government officials. Our program is different. The women have no connections whatsoever with influential people.

Do women in PNG have things in common with women in Australia?

They have a lot in common. Being women, we all have problems to do with everyday living. We have to struggle twice as hard to be recognised, to be accepted and to contribute something towards development of our society.

Desley, you've mentioned nutrition. What are some of the other women's health issues?

Water. Our women have to walk such a long distance to collect water. And they are carrying children and food as well. Water may be 10 kilometres away. It is too much, it is very tiring. They limp back. One of the women in our program is building water tanks and pumps.

Where do women have their babies?

Usually women have babies in their villages. We have just started training village midwives. But there is still a very high rate of children dying. It is not uncommon for the mother to die also.

If there are complications, what happens?

The baby just dies. I knew a woman who was going to have twins. She had one twin in the village but the other one wouldn't come out. It was a two-hour drive from the village to the hospital and the second baby died on the way. The woman was just lucky that she didn't die too.

Is the government expanding health services?

The services the Health Department provides are very limited. We have worked along with the Health Department in just one district to get the women in for a period of two or three weeks to learn basic first aid.

The women took the first aid box back to the village. Soon the supplies ran out. The Health Department won't take the responsibility to send us more. It comes back to us women, and it's a very hard thing. Sometimes we go to get more supplies. Sometimes we don't because of transport. It means walking if you have to.

There are so many cuts and many people have very ugly ulcers on their skin. There's no transport. People don't own cars. They don't want to spend hours travelling by foot so they don't go for treatment. They use traditional plant remedies for sores, diarrhoea, backaches, infections, and even abortion.

If the woman wants to have an abortion, what happens?

It's not talked about very often because abortion is illegal in PNG. But what the woman will do is go to another woman in town who everybody knows. Word has quietly gotten around about who does abortions. So a woman just goes and says, 'I need an abortion.' Certain leaves and flowers are used.

What methods of contraception are used?

We have a program in our network on family planning but the Catholic Church is against it. So a lot of women are afraid to come to our program and their husbands also don't like it. What that means is that women aren't using any contraception at all and have nine, ten or eleven children.

Even in town it's very rare for women to buy condoms. They might feel ashamed. If it's a young, single woman and she goes to the hospital to ask for contraception, people will tell stories about her. It used to be a very bad thing for a single woman to have sexual relations. It's still strict.

In our culture, if a woman stays single, people start to say, 'She's funny, how come she's not married?' Although now it's starting to be more acceptable.

That attitude is common in many countries and here in Australia as well.

Are sexually transmitted diseases an issue?

Yes, but people are ashamed. It's taboo. And it's a very big problem now. Our village women won't talk about it. Even women in town won't talk about it.

What are marriage customs like in Papua New Guinea?

In Papua New Guinea, different groups have different customs. In East Sepik men are allowed to have more than one wife. They can have as many as four wives. I have known businessmen who have four wives in Papua New Guinea and East Sepik. The so-called big men show their riches by having more than one wife. Of course, women cannot have more than one husband.

Husbands are often beating their wives too. It's not unusual to hear women screaming.

With such problems to overcome, can you tell me something about your overall vision for PNG women?

I am glad that our government in Papua New Guinea has recognised women and wants our women to have an equal contribution and say in our development. It's the seventh point of the Equal Plan.

But in reality there are very few resources and a lot of difficulty trying to gain financial assistance from the government. I think it comes back to us women. We have to really show the government that we can do something, and that women need to be educated and equal for the good of the country.

Part II

Some Facts of Life

The IUD
A cautionary tale

Roma Cusack interviewed by Rose Sorger

Roma, I remember talking to you about eight years ago and being horrified to hear your account of the effects of an IUD insertion. Could you think back and tell me what happened?

I had a problem with pain in the hip in 1981. At that stage I was 41 and I thought I'd go and have my mid-life check. I went to a GP and asked could I have an x-ray on my hip to get that sorted out. I had a phone call a couple of days later from the receptionist who said, 'The doctor would like to talk to you about your IUD.' 'I haven't got an IUD,' I said. 'I lost it eight years ago.' 'Well it looks like a Dalkon Shield,' she said. I went in to see the x-ray and discuss it. There it was—very clear on the x-ray. The IUD had perforated my uterus and lodged in my hip.

The background to this is that I'd had a baby in April 1972. About six weeks later in May or June 1972, I'd had a Dalkon Shield inserted on the advice of my then gynaecologist/obstetrician who was supposedly one of the top men in Melbourne. I didn't realise how new it was then, but it was obviously the best thing since sliced bread. I didn't want to go on the pill as I was breastfeeding. The day that it was inserted I was expecting to be measured only. But he said, 'We might as well do it now'. I experienced this most excruciating pain, much worse than childbirth. I practically fainted. I walked out of the room and the nurse said, 'You look terrible, would you like a cup of tea and to sit down?'

I had a number of stomach cramps and sharp pains. I'd later rung the gynaecologist and been told that it took a little while to settle down, which it did, and I felt nothing further. I don't remember any other symptoms such as bleeding.

If you talk to women and read the related literature, it appears that there are often no ongoing recognisable symptoms after perforation of the uterus by an IUD.

Yes—I didn't feel anything further and I didn't get pregnant, so I assumed it was working. Two and a half years after that first baby, I wanted to have another baby. I was 32. In September or October of 1973, I went back to the gynaecologist to have the IUD removed. He couldn't find it and thought I'd probably expelled it. He sent me immediately to have an x-ray to see if it was visible. It wasn't, so he just assumed that I'd expelled it. I don't know what that x-ray consisted of but I assume now that either the IUD didn't show or it was an x-ray of a specific part of the uterus only.

I remember thinking, if not saying, 'How can I lose an IUD and not know it?' In fact, I must have voiced it because I remember someone saying, 'Oh yes, they can just come out.' Then in 1981 when I had my hip x-ray it showed the IUD.

I couldn't believe it, although I saw the x-ray. The IUD was there, clear as a bell.

Where was it located, Roma?

Well, I subsequently had an ultrasound and I was told again I was in the hands of the best man in Melbourne. He couldn't locate it specifically enough for anyone to make a decision to go in after it. It was outside the uterus, probably embedded. I had an internal examination to check that, and it was one of the most revolting experiences I have ever had—horrible, painful. My feelings were quite mixed. I was shocked and angry because I wasn't expecting this at all. I thought the IUD had gone in 1973.

I was working in the information centre at the Royal Women's Hospital when I first spoke to you. You told me you really needed information about your situation and asked, 'Can this happen?' I remember we went through all the literature, and you then felt you had more to go on.

Yes, I knew that I was like most people in doctors' hands and that without some unbiased professional help I'd get nowhere. I didn't want to move until I felt I had that backing. So then I thought, I'm not going back to that man who did it to me, so where *do* I go to, who do I turn to? I don't think it occurred to me to go back to my GP. I wanted another specialist.

I thought of the Doctors' Reform Society because I thought they might be the straightest with me. So I phoned and said to the doctor who answered, 'I'm a very angry lady and I want to go to someone I can trust. Who would you send your wife to?' He gave me the name of someone. I also spoke to a lawyer friend of mine and decided that I was going to have a witness this time. So I took my husband.

This doctor was very understanding. I also told him I was very angry and why. He was very nice and I felt quite comfortable and confident with him. He answered all my questions and made the visit a full hour. I didn't feel rushed at all.

He did an internal and said, 'If you can bear it—it's to ascertain that the IUD really isn't in the uterus.' He inserted some long object which was awful because it caused contractions just like labour. After that I thought I was going to be sick.

All of these examinations were without any sort of pain relief or much explanation by the sound of things.

Well, he said, 'It will be uncomfortable but if you can stand it, it would be easier to get it over with.' So I did. I don't know about my pain threshold. I'd always thought it was low but I think now it's probably pretty high. Anyway that settled the question that there was no IUD in the uterus.

Then the doctor suggested that I have an ultrasound, because he wanted to be precise and sure about where it was. He presented some choices. He suggested it was probably embedded in tissue and just sitting there, as he said, 'like a piece of shrapnel'. If I wasn't presenting any symptoms it was probably best to leave things alone.

That's an interesting analogy.

Yes, beautiful—the after-effects of war, with me as a battleground! The other choice was to go in after it. He said, 'It's very messy in there, not like the textbooks. It's very slippery and very close to the main artery which goes down your leg. Avoid any surgery like that if you can.'

The ultrasound person couldn't find it clearly. He thought he saw it but he wasn't absolutely certain. On the basis of all this the doctor advised me to do nothing, just to leave it there. He said he was 99 per cent sure it wasn't connected to my hip pain and I think that's probably right.

How do you feel about the fact that you were advised to keep this piece of foreign material in your body and that it is still there today? Does it bother you?

Well, I don't like it. I tend not to think about it very much. But every now and again the press will have a statement about it. The American compensation case, of which I'm a part, will make the news on the television or there will be a special on an IUD, and it will come back.

I'm usually a fairly easy-going sort of person. I really don't make too much fuss about anything. But this does make me very, very angry and I feel the hairs on the back of my neck crinkle. I think of it as a sort of time bomb in my body, even though I know other people are walking around with things like shrapnel in them.

The huge difference of course is that this is a method of contraception that was presented to women as being safe and preventing pregnancy— not harmful.

Oh yes, nobody wants this foreign body. The anger doesn't go away. It's almost inexpressible. I didn't go back to the original gynaecologist because I thought I might strangle him. And the professional position for the second-opinion gynaecologist was obviously difficult because he didn't say anything about the first guy.

There are some people who consider that in the large majority of perforations of the uterus, the practitioner has had a poor technique, that a sound [measure] hasn't been used, for example, to determine the size of the uterine cavity. Was there any mention of incompetence?

No, but then again I didn't ask questions that I thought might embarrass him. I was more concerned with the situation and what we were going to do about it. My feelings about the first gynaecologist were so very strong that I didn't want to put my current one in a difficult position. I could see that would be hard for him.

Did you ever try to get your medical records?

Well, I subsequently found myself part of the litigation in the United States through the Office of the Public Interest Advocacy Centre in Sydney. They sought records from the original doctor. I gave them his address.

I did think quite seriously of suing him, but I was quickly dissuaded from that position by legal people I knew who said, 'Don't bother, you won't win.' There were difficulties getting all the records. Some aren't kept after seven years.

Strangely, a friend of mine who had a loop inserted by the same gynaecologist who inserted my IUD went to have an x-ray. A clever radiologist noticed that she'd had her tubes tied and wanted to know why they were tied when she still had a Lippes Loop! Anyway within a fortnight she was in hospital and had it out. In that intervening fortnight it had moved from one side of her body to the other.

She then said to me, 'You can't go overseas with that in you. You've got to have it out.' I went to the GP and said, 'What if I'm on some Greek mountain and something goes wrong?' 'Don't worry, you'll be fine,' he said. I insisted, 'Come on, what could happen?' 'Well, there is a million-to-one chance,' he told me, 'that it could perforate your bowel.' 'How would I know?' I asked. 'You'll know,' he said, 'you'd be writhing on the floor.'

So no one had discussed with you at either the original insertion or after it was found outside the uterus, what the complications were in regard to an IUD?

Oh no. I can remember recently seeing some of this on the Copper 7 IUD TV program. I remember after the second baby thinking I'd have another IUD, not knowing it was still there of course. They thought the Copper 7 was the greatest thing. They were saying, 'This is the one we've been waiting for.' But my husband said, 'No. No one knows what copper is going to do inside your body. You're not going to do it.' But could you imagine if I'd had the Copper 7 as well as the Dalkon Shield floating around!

What a thought! So Roma, you were a part of the 1981 US National Women's Health Network class action lawsuit against the A. H. Robins pharmaceutical company?

Right.

They were seeking a worldwide recall of the Shield and estimated that there were 50 000 women in the US and 500 000 women in other countries around the world still with the Dalkon Shield inside them. It gives some idea of the dimension of it all.

They were still inserting it some time after this, even after a program on television about three years ago. It really made my blood boil, because there was a doctor in Melbourne still inserting it in Turkish women in 1984.

And yet it came off the market in the States in 1974. Often these dangerous devices and harmful substances targeted for women continue to be marketed outside the USA or country of origin, particularly in Third World countries.

Yes, but there is no excuse for this to happen in Australia. I also saw in this program on the Copper 7, a Robins company public relations person, a woman, God help us, describe it all as a 'ball game' and that some were going to win and some were going to lose. This is incredible, because many women had injuries much worse than mine.

You've kept a keen eye on all this. Do you know of the problems encountered by other women?

Oh yes. Women have had infected uteruses, septic miscarriages, to say nothing of the trauma that goes with all of this. If *I'm* experiencing anger with no physical symptoms, what must it be like for those women? It must be horrific.

I've known women who have found their uterus to be full of pus and have gone on to develop chronic pelvic infections, and associated fertility problems. This has absolutely changed how they felt as women, along with seriously impairing their health.

In the papers I get from the class action, there are litigants who are not the prime sufferer. There is clearly room for the partners to put in claims because of the effect on relationships. Sexual lives are interrupted or fraught.

Was it any help to you to share your feelings and the other information you had with other women?

For my friend and I, it was particularly helpful to sound off against the same gynaecologist. We thought it was too much of a coincidence.

I contacted the original gynaecologist to have a copy of my records sent to my current GP because the gynaecologist probably wouldn't have sent them to me. I don't think Freedom of Information covers private doctors. The GP was sent a copy of my records and I went to see him. He wouldn't give me a copy but said, 'I'll read it to you.' In my records it was written that when I'd gone back to have the IUD taken out, I'd been seen by a locum. 'What? I didn't see a locum,' I told the GP. But I still had a doubt in my mind about that—such is their power, even over someone like me, who'd gone through a lot of the anger and been politicised by the whole thing. I now know that I wasn't wrong about this, but the GP's copy of my record shows I saw a locum and I was horrified.

Also imagine, Roma, women who have limited language skills, women who are in Third World countries where they have no information of any sort.

God knows what happens to them! Also, I meant to mention that when I made the phone call to the original gynaecologist's office, I was shaking because I didn't want to say too much, just get the records to the GP. I don't know how the Dalkon Shield came up but the receptionist asked, 'Are you one of those women who had a problem with it?' I said, 'It's still inside me.' She laughed. I couldn't believe it! I was shaking with rage. I think she reported this to her boss. I think this is why the records were falsified. I don't know how one deals with this.

It is a problem but more women are getting to know their rights now. We have women's health action groups and services. Mind you, many doctors are extremely wary about all this and have a strong dislike of women who collectively take up these issues. What else have you felt about this experience, Roma?

Well, I guess apart from the emotional effect, it's been very helpful to be part of a large group of women across the world who are taking action on this, to have some acknowledgement and compensation made. There are billions of dollars involved. The only thing wrong is all the forms you have to fill in. It's never-ending.

All these years later it's still going on?

Yes. I had it put in in 1972—it's seventeen years! It's a long time to be dealing with something—which they thought was a miracle. I'd go for the diaphragm any day.

There is such a lack of research information about contraceptive methods and their effects. The long- and short-term risks are not adequately assessed or explained.

Yet one assumes they have been approved, that all sorts of stringent tests have been conducted, and that it's only then that products are released into the market. In fact, the Robins company's own documents apparently show that their research on the Dalkon Shield was invalid and inadequate and the Food and Drug Administration in the US accepted Robins' evidence.

The doctor who designed the Shield promoted it through a prominent medical journal and other forums. This also gave it considerable credibility.

There is no end to it, is there? It certainly politicised me in regard to feminism. I view the world differently now.

Roma, thank you for the interview. I realise it brings it all to the forefront again for you.

Postscript

The abbreviation IUD stands for intrauterine device. The device is usually made of metal or plastic. It is inserted into the uterus to prevent pregnancy. IUDs come in various sizes and shapes and are made by different companies. Some of the brand names of IUDs are the Nova-T, the Copper 7, sold as Gravigard in Australia, the Multi-Load CU250 and the Dalkon Shield.

It is not known exactly how the IUD works as a contraceptive, only that the IUD makes it difficult for a fertilised egg to be implanted in the uterus and develop. IUDs, although highly reliable as a contraceptive, are not 100 per cent effective.

There are several risks associated with IUDs. A majority of women who have never been pregnant suffer severe pain and bleeding if they use an IUD, especially during their periods, but sometimes between periods as well.

Although the IUD obstructs a fertilised egg from growing in the uterus, the fertilised egg may become implanted outside the uterus, in the fallopian tubes, for example. Four to 5 per cent of women who become pregnant while using an IUD have one of these ectopic pregnancies.

Another problem with IUDs is that they increase the risk of women getting an infection in the uterus or fallopian tubes by three to five times compared with women who do not use IUDs. This type of infection is known as pelvic inflammatory disease (PID). One in six women who have had PID become infertile because of scarring and narrowing of the tubes.

An IUD can also perforate the uterus or be expelled from the uterus, sometimes lodging in other parts of the pelvic region. Although rare, IUD complications have even resulted in death. Two Australian women have died from IUD complications.

Between 1971 and 1975 the A. H. Robins pharmaceutical company distributed over four million Dalkon Shield IUDs in 80 countries. At the time when A. H. Robins put the Dalkon Shield on the market, the US Food and Drug Administration was not required to approve devices. This has since changed.

Many women have been damaged by the Dalkon Shield. The design and fibre used in making a part of the device leaves women vulnerable to infection. In Australia alone, over 7000 women have sued Robins for the harmful effects they suffered from the Dalkon Shield. In February 1989 a woman in New South Wales became the first Australian to receive compensation from Robins. Fortunately, unlike others, she did not have permanent damage from the IUD. But she waited fifteen years for the nominal payment of $860 from Robins.

The Dalkon Shield is no longer prescribed for women in Australia. The Copper 7 IUD, which has also caused similar problems for women, was withdrawn from the United States market in 1986. It is still sold and recommended in Australia under the name of Gravigard.

The choice of which IUDs stay on the market is partly dependent on the power of the corporations or agencies that produce them. Why was the Dalkon Shield, for example, singled out for criticism? The World Health Organisation has a contract for manufacturing the Copper 7 IUD in developing countries. Other large pharmaceuticals have also carved out an IUD market. Perhaps the relatively small A. H. Robins company was a threat to other manufacturers' profits. They may not have been sorry to see a competitor, who was trying to enter the big league, being attacked.

References

Adams, Jad 'Who stood to gain on the Dalkon Shield?' *New Scientist* 26 September 1985, pp. 74–5

Conley, Jennifer 'Dalkon claimants will continue action' *The Age* 21 July 1988, p. 16

Miller, Benjamin and Keane, Claire *Encyclopedia and Dictionary of Medicine, Nursing, and Allied Health* Sydney: W. B. Saunders, 1987, pp. 657–8

Mintz, Morton *At Any Cost: Women, Profits, and the Dalkon Shield* New York: Pantheon, 1985

Wheatley, Jane 'The Copper 7 Controversy: "I Should Have Asked More Questions, Made More Fuss" ' *The Australian Women's Weekly* February 1989, pp. 28–30

Gender politics and AIDS

Judith Jones

Are we as women at risk of becoming infected with the HIV virus? Is it even a question which needs to be asked? I believe that we must raise and attempt to answer it if we are to be successful in preventing any further spread of the HIV virus, because an important part of prevention involves challenging the perception that women, in general, are not at risk.

It is not difficult to see how that myth has arisen. In the West, AIDS appears to be definitely a disease of males. As of mid-May 1989, of the total of 1334 people diagnosed with AIDS, only 46 are female. Of those, 23 were infected by blood transfusions, ten from heterosexual activity, seven from sharing needles and syringes, and six cases are still under investigation or the transmission category is unknown. In Australia, 26 women had died from AIDS by mid-May 1989.

While on the face of it these numbers don't seem to suggest any significant risks for women, figures from other industrialised countries give more cause for concern. For example, in the United States, 8.6 per cent of people diagnosed as having AIDS are female, and in Europe as a whole, the figure is 10.2 per cent. Approximately half these women became infected through intravenous drug use. The next most common way was from heterosexual contact with an infected male.

In Australia, where infection from contaminated blood transfusions and products has been eliminated, the highest risks are linked with unprotected intercourse and sharing drug-using equipment with a person carrying the virus.

Theoretically, the risks involved in these two activities are the same for females as for males. But are they really equal? Yes and no. In some ways, risk factors like sharing fixes and intercourse don't seem to differentiate between the sexes. But in heterosexual intercourse women are more vulnerable to infection, because of the amount of semen left in their bodies.

As well there are more subtle, less visible factors which markedly increase the vulnerability of women. These are issues to do with women's socialisation and sexual politics.

All women are subject to social and cultural factors or conditioning that place us in a less powerful social and sexual position in society. It does not matter whether we are single or partnered, workers in the sex industry or not. Women are at risk, not only because of what we do, but also as a result of how others behave, because of who we are and how we are viewed by others. As long as we are seen primarily as sex objects, as long as we are less powerful than men socially or economically, as long as we lack practice in assertion and negotiation, we are at increased risk of infection with HIV or any other disease which is passed from person to person by sexual activity.

Why is this so? Women get HIV sexually from men. Not only do very many more men than women carry the HIV virus, especially in Australia, but both females and males are trained from early childhood to believe that the role of women involves catering to the emotional and sexual needs of men. The very existence of the sex industry illustrates that. Men have sexual needs and women's bodies are used in the satisfying of those needs. The acceptance of this dynamic underpins both marriage and prostitution. Moreover, the notion of 'sex' is equated with intercourse, with its associated risks for women. Without doubt, in the heterosexual community, the campaign for safer sex will be successful if men can be persuaded to wear condoms, and to realise that non-penetrative sex (i.e. sex which doesn't involve insertion of the penis) can also be sexy, satisfying and masculine.

Very often women are unable or unwilling to say no to potentially risky sexual practices because we are economically dependent on men. This is a very real issue for some women in the sex industry, whether working independently or for male management.

Unemployed and impoverished women experience the feelings of powerlessness and vulnerability which can result from economic hardship and the consequent loss of self-esteem. Even a cursory socio-economic analysis of the AIDS figures from the United States shows that this is primarily a disease of the poor, the alienated and the disenfranchised; and all over the world, there are more women in those categories than men.

Another dimension of the vulnerability of women with regard to HIV and other STDs lies in the extent of their emotional dependence on men and in their understanding of the meaning of love. Many women, perhaps especially the young, derive a much-needed sense of personal value from their sexual partnership with a man, but lack the personal skills to negotiate in terms of their own health needs.

For example, we know there are young women who share needles and syringes with their male sexual partners because sharing demonstrates the emotional bond between them. In the same way, we know that while prostitutes may protect themselves from risk of sexual infection while working, they often don't use condoms or practice safe sex with their regular partner.

Another risk to women is the widespread acceptance, at least at some deep psychological level, of a double standard of sexual behaviour, particularly when this behaviour is kept secret. How many women are unwittingly vulnerable to infection because of the unsuspected and undisclosed risky activities of their sexual mate?

Of particular concern are the women whose partners, unknown to them, engage in covert sex with other men. Prevailing community values, beliefs, and in some places laws, with regard to homosexuality and intravenous drug use ensure that there is the threat of total rejection of anyone who admits to these behaviours. Many of these men may be too afraid to tell their female partner of the danger to her health; altogether, there must be many unsuspecting women in this kind of hazardous situation.

While as yet there may be no substantial transmission of the HIV virus to women in Australia, I have argued that there are powerful social structures and expectations which compound the dangers for women in already potentially hazardous areas. Solutions in this area are not simple; the factors involved—socialisation, economics, sexual interaction—are powerful and complex. Nonetheless, it is essential that we acknowledge the potential risk of HIV infection for all people who are involved in risky activities, and that we recognise the additional vulnerability of many women.

Ultimately, we must work to strengthen the social and sexual position of women in our society, to address female unemployment and poverty, to endorse the importance of the total health and well-being of women, and to increase the ability of women to be articulate, assertive and confident about themselves and their place in the world.

Thus, while HIV presents us all with a myriad of challenges, surely one of the greatest is the need to challenge societal assumptions about the ways in which women and men relate, and to address the inequities of sexual politics which affect every aspect of the lives of women.

Encore

Two women at menopause

Helen Myles and Deborah Davison interviewed by Kathy Wilson

You've been friends for some time and you both experienced menopause at roughly the same time.

Helen: I was the first one to go into menopause. When I was 47 I missed three periods in a row. At the same time I began to experience hot flushes. For me, this is a tingly sort of feeling throughout my body, with a really hot feeling in my face, followed by sweating.

After three or four months my period came back. For the next year I had normal periods again and no flushes. Then suddenly the periods stopped again and the flushes started. It's now over eighteen months since I menstruated but I have continued to have hot flushes. I think I'm through menopause, but I don't know how long the flushes will last. At first they were really regular. Some days I would feel one every couple of hours. They would wake me in the middle of the night. I'd be in such a sweat and throw off the bedclothes for a few minutes until I cooled down. The flushes I have now are less intense and don't last as long.

I tend to tell people with me when I'm having one of these flushes, because it feels so obvious to me and I imagine it must be noticeable to others. I once told my mother and she said, 'I know, I can see your face going pink', and that's how it feels—like a blush with moisture.

Deborah: My experience was different from Helen's. For one thing I am ten years younger. I have a history of very easy periods that lasted just two or three days and were fairly light. Suddenly I started having very heavy periods that lasted longer and were much more painful. I went to a doctor, but basically I put up with it. Then I went for three to four months without a period but had no hot flushes or any other symptom. A few months later I went to the doctor again because I started having hot flushes. I didn't call them

45

that though—they were panic attacks to me. The periods continued not to come, a funny way of putting it, but that is how it felt. Every month would tick by and I would still not get a period. Then one day I had slight bleeding, not a real period, and that caused the doctor some concern. I had a D and C but there was nothing wrong and still no periods. That's another difference between Helen and me—my period stopped before I started to have hot flushes.

Did you realise you may have been starting menopause?

Deborah: That wasn't in my mind and it wasn't in the doctor's mind to begin with either, because I was only in my late thirties. I did go to another doctor then, a doctor who I was told would be more sympathetic and who had more knowledge in this area. She said, 'Well perhaps this is menopause, or perhaps it is anxiety and stress.' Since I was still quite young I thought maybe it was some kind of emotional reaction.

Helen: Whereas I was expecting it. As soon as I didn't get my period, I thought, 'This is menopause.' I immediately accepted it as a time of change.

How did you feel about being in a period of change? What did you think about?

Helen: I felt OK about it. I thought I would deal with it as I had menstruation, childbirth and breastfeeding—the other aspects of my reproductive life. I had no problems with menstruation and I had two fairly short and easy births. So my experience of things reproductive was that they just came about and you went through them. I think that's how I approached menopause. I felt quite good. I was pleased to be finishing my periods.

Did you miss bleeding?

Helen: No, not at all.

Deborah: Once again I am vastly different because I felt in absolute turmoil, very depressed by it and very confused. I kept shouting to myself, 'I'm too young. What's happening to me? This isn't fair. I don't want to deal with this. I'm not prepared. I haven't read enough. I haven't talked to enough people. I'm not ready.'

I felt a sense of loss that was hard to explain. I didn't want another child, so it wasn't about a lost opportunity or anything like that, although I did question this. Maybe I really did want another baby.

Perhaps a woman who experiences very bad periods would be glad to see the end of them. I didn't experience bad periods and I did experience this sense of loss when they stopped. There were times when I was crying and grief stricken.

What other changes happened physically and emotionally?

Deborah: It seemed like I was constantly either too hot or too cold. Dryness of the vagina was a real shock. Even though I had known about it as a symptom, when it actually happened to me it was very difficult.

An interesting aspect of menopause is trying to make connections between the different things that are happening to you. I had headaches but I didn't know if they were because of anxiety or because of the menopause. I was feeling a loss of sexual libido. I was also depressed and insecure. I had to ask myself which were causes, which were effects.

Helen: I asked those cause-and-effect questions too, even though I didn't experience the dry vagina you are talking about. In fact, I experienced almost the exact opposite—an upsurge in my libido. That was all mixed up with wanting to form a new sexual relationship. So both physical and huge emotional changes were happening in my life. I experienced enormous confusion about all these new thoughts and feelings. I constantly asked myself if wanting to leave my partner of 25 years and feeling sexually aroused by someone else was only because I was going through menopause, and that if I waited just a little while it would all go away. In other words, my confusion was not to do with the loss of my bodily function but to do with changing in other ways—wanting to move outward in a way that I had never done before. I was reminded of Margaret Mead's expression 'post-menopausal zest', which sums up where I am now.

Were your relationships also affected, Deborah?

Deborah: Oh disastrously, because it seems to me that a partner can be tolerant, loving, tender and understanding for only so long. There is a limit. Through all this I was finding it so hard to deal with that I couldn't talk about it, whereas in the past I had been able to talk about sex.

Also, I didn't know how long I was going to have hot flushes. This was not helped by the fact that books say it can go on for several years. In fact, that's what I've been experiencing for eighteen months plus. It's hard to say to my partner, 'Look, just hang around for a few years and I will be all right again.'

There was some stress in your life related to other things at this time wasn't there? How can you separate the variables of all the things that are happening in your life from the menopause?

Deborah: It has been a very stressful time for me. But I can't help feeling that when I had been going through hard times before, I had a reserve to draw on. I was able to cope and thought, 'Yes, OK it is a bad day.' What I've experienced going through menopause is that I seem to have very little reserve. I don't think, 'Oh, it's just because I'm down today and I'll be all right tomorrow. All I need is a long weekend.' That sort of positive feeling is not there because I don't know how long it will take me to get through menopause. I have an irrational sense that this is somehow all my fault or a weakness.

Once I saw myself as a sexual person. That was part of my identity. I also saw myself as a person who coped with the rough and tumble—down one day, up the next—competent. Now my confidence has been shattered. I know it sounds pretty bad, but I also know that some women have an even worse experience.

Have you talked to other people about this? Menopause was once something that wasn't spoken about. I think I know when my mother went through menopause, but she certainly didn't tell me. I don't know if she spoke to others in the family. How was it for you and the people you live with?

Deborah: My mum didn't tell me about her experiences. I don't feel we could talk even now except in a very superficial way. I don't feel too upset about that because that's the nature of our relationship.

The reactions of some of my friends distressed me. They laughed and joked when I mentioned menopause because I'm still quite young. They said things like, 'Oh no, it can't be the menopause. Don't be silly. There is something else happening.' It got to the point where I found I wasn't talking to people about it because I was so upset by this response of disbelief. Maybe menopause is still a taboo subject and their laughter was covering up their sense of uneasiness about discussing it. Few women wanted to talk with me about it. Helen and I were able to talk with understanding because we were both going through it at the same time.

Certainly women in their late thirties are not thinking about it and I find this quite alarming. Because if I had thought about it before it happened to me I would have been much better prepared emotionally, physically and socially. I think there is an apathy about menopause. There aren't even any good jokes about it.

Helen: My mother didn't tell me at the time about her menopause, but as adults we have talked about it. When my hot flushes became very frequent I rang my mother and asked her to tell me what happened to her when she went through menopause. 'Oh, I had hot flushes. I used to get them all the time,' she said. I asked her what they felt like and she reported to me exactly what I was feeling. She said she had them for quite a while, but that was the only physical symptom she had. Her experience seemed similar to mine and that was really comforting to me. It helped me accept it easily.

Did you talk to your children about it?

Helen: Yes, I told them I was going through menopause and about the physical and some of the emotional changes I was experiencing. My kids just accepted it because we have discussed those sorts of things all along.

Deborah: I don't think my daughter could connect with what I was saying, although she did try to understand. I obviously talked with her about it but I don't think it was easy for her. She was going through puberty at the same time and I think that is an interesting dynamic that happens in families. Often a mother can be going through menopause at the same time as a daughter is going through puberty. My daughter seemed to be managing puberty better than I was managing menopause. That's for sure.

Helen: I felt I was sometimes experiencing similar things to my daughter. She was seventeen, and moving into adulthood. I felt as if I was going into another stage of my life too. It seemed to have more significance than just the physical changes. It was like the end of an era. My kids were grown up and my body's capacity to produce children was gone. It was really a definitive time. One part of my life was ending and I was moving into something different. It felt as if I had a chance to open up, to be free, physically, sexually and emotionally.

Deborah: Some people say that how women feel during menopause is partly in their heads, or socially and culturally influenced. But the physical symptoms are real, no matter what age a woman is or what culture she comes from. Women of all classes or races may experience hot flushes or anxiety.

But there does seem to be a social context for menopause too. Currently it is becoming a little more talked about, yet in some of the literature, research and publicity it is being described as an illness that has to be treated with hormones, for example.

Helen: I think you are right. Menopause is the last frontier of women's reproduction to be exploited. The population is aging and drug companies no doubt see a lucrative market. If menopause is promoted as an illness, the pharmaceutical industry can profit from selling hormones. In addition, women have become much more assertive regarding their health rights in relation to menstruation, contraception and childbirth, but the medical profession hasn't been confronted in the same way yet about menopause.

I want to say that I haven't at any time felt that I needed to be 'treated'. I was pretty sure that my hot flushes were a natural phenomonen so I didn't go to a doctor.

But Deborah, you did use medication.

Yes, I had hormonal therapy which was helpful although it did cause side effects. For example, my breasts swelled to the size they were when I was pregnant and felt painful. There is some debate about our bodies' need for oestrogen. The fact that I am going to live for years with lowered oestrogen in my body is perhaps a problem. You still have some oestrogen being produced, though. The issue for younger people is whether that is enough over a long period of time. This is my doctor's explanation for why somebody of my age needs oestrogen replacement therapy. But this doesn't answer why some older women are taking hormones.

When you started having oestrogen, did you know what to ask to get the information you needed to make the decision?

Deborah: I went to the doctor several times before I decided to have it. I did some reading and asked other women who'd opted for oestrogen therapy what they thought.

I still find it quite complicated and have mixed views. I feel a bit frustrated that I can't come down on one side or the other and say, 'Yes, I'm pro it' or 'I'm anti it'. But once I got the low dosage that suited me I felt better. Certainly it helps the anxiety aspect of hot flushes.

So you have been through different dosages, very similar to women taking the pill?

That's right. And the lower dose seems all right. There are no side effects that I am aware of, but who knows?

Helen: Do you have some idea of how long you are going to be on it?

Deborah: The doctor said for ever, but I don't feel comfortable with the thought of being on oestrogen replacement therapy for the rest of my life. Yet I don't want to develop osteoporosis with bones that break on me when I'm elderly. If one of the functions of oestrogen is that it helps absorb calcium then I guess I must take it. But I wish there was more research being done on whether taking hormones is really necessary because right now you hear conflicting reports and don't know what to do. I don't know if there is much funding for research for preventing osteoporosis rather than 'treating' it.

What about the way in which women are described? It seems to me that if women do something a bit different or a little unusual you hear things like, 'Oh, she's going through the change of life', as if it was a period of madness.

Helen: That doubt hung over me. People told me menopause was to blame for the new and different way I was thinking and acting. I denied it vehemently, but it was hard to remain firm in my resolve that I was changing as a person and not 'suffering' a psychological symptom.

At first I was very defensive, but then I tried to think about the two being linked. Perhaps they were. I don't know. I don't think it really mattered in the end whether they were. I was feeling different. It was happening to me and whether the changes I have mentioned were caused by menopause or not they have remained consistent and strong for two years now.

Deborah: In many ways it is like so many areas when women say, 'This is how I feel' or 'This is what I am going to do' or 'This is what I want or need'. It is often disregarded or derided by people around her, husbands, lovers, children, parents or friends. It seems that menopause brings that out in stark relief—perceptions of women as mad or bad.

I really needed a group of women to talk with, especially younger women who were going through menopause. But I wasn't feeling assertive enough to go and find that.

How did you manage at work?

Deborah: There were times when I'd be on the phone and get a flush and I couldn't continue the conversation. Some women working around me were sympathetic and compassionate but I still felt I had to hide it.

Helen: I did actually tell people about it. I still do. Just this week

I went into a meeting with men and women and as I sat down I was conscious that I was having a hot flush and starting to sweat. I explained it to the assembled group as I dabbed my face. I don't suppose they knew whether I was being serious or making a joke.

Deborah: I wasn't able to do that, because a few times when I did, people would look at me quizzically and say, 'What, hot flushes at your age?' They'd laugh and say I was mad which was exactly what I was feeling.

Helen: Whereas perhaps because of my age people accept it from me. They don't ask me a lot of questions. They usually don't say anything. Perhaps they're so stunned at the mention of menopause that they don't know how to react.

Deborah: We haven't learnt what to say or do when a woman says, 'I'm having a hot flush.' Is there a response? Do you want a response? Maybe you do, maybe you don't.

Helen: I don't really want them to say anything, but I sometimes need to explain what I am experiencing.

Deborah: But if you do want a response, you can be sure most people haven't learned through social interaction what to say. For example, when someone sneezes everybody knows to say, 'Bless you.'

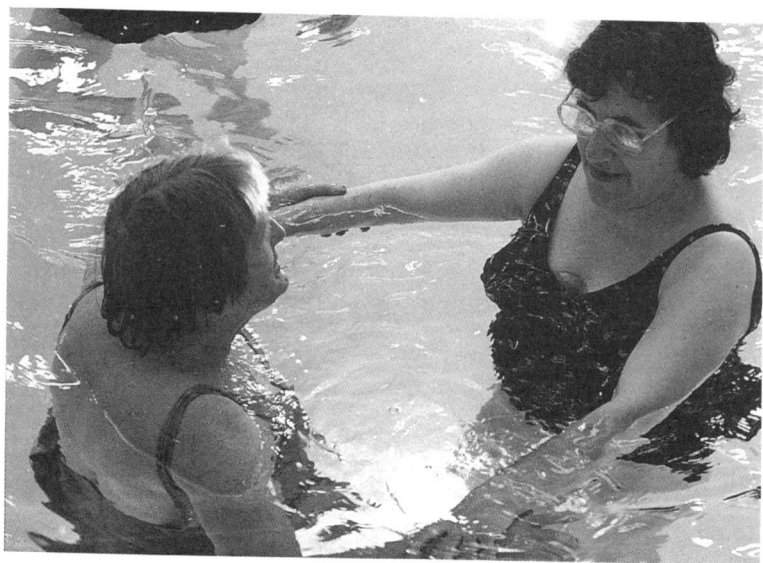

Water exercises, Joyce Agee, 1989

Not too young to know

Susan Wright interviewed by Rose Sorger

Sue, you conducted a study of young secondary students across Victoria. Could you tell me how it got going?

The study was initiated by the Royal Australian College of Obstetricians and Gynaecologists who were concerned about young women's ignorance of their sexual and reproductive health, for instance in regard to cervical cancer. The aim of the study was to find out what information young women required.

I was employed as the research officer. I felt that rather than always talking to health professionals and teachers about what young people need to know, we might go to the source directly and ask them what their concerns were.

How many young people did you talk to and in what way did you gather your information?

We talked to 1351 young people all in Year 10, which is about the fourteen-and-a-half to fifteen-and-a-half year age group. We had a true random sample of Victorian schools going across all systems—state, Catholic and other independents, metropolitan and non-metropolitan. We worked on a questionnaire which contained many little stories, little vignettes, to outline certain scenarios and we asked students to comment on what they thought was the best way to act for this imaginary couple. At the end of the questionnaire I asked for volunteers for groups of up to twenty students for discussions with me and we interviewed well over 500 students in this way.

Did these young men and women have difficulty talking about sexuality?

Not at all. They were amazingly easy to talk to. But at no stage did I make any question personal such as asking, 'What is your behaviour?' or 'Have you had sex?' I talked in much more general terms.

Is it your impression that if you had been more personal it would have been difficult to get certain information?

Most likely, and the greatest difficulty would have been to get honest information. People would have answered the way they thought they ought to.

So what were some of the main findings, Sue?

Students knew a bit in some areas and then there were great gaps in knowledge. They may have heard about sexually transmitted diseases, for example—of course everybody has heard about AIDS and condoms—but when it came to the much more common sexually transmitted diseases like chlamydia, students were almost completely ignorant and particularly about sexually transmitted diseases which have no symptoms. These of course are the most dangerous for girls because they lead to pelvic inflammatory disease and infertility in many cases, and students know very little about this.

Did you find that students had difficulty gaining information about health?

Yes. This was what I personally consider the most important finding of the study—the difficulty that still exists for young people to get accurate information. Right across the board, young people talk to other friends, and they are the first ones to admit that friends don't necessarily present them with good information because they also haven't got the facts. For instance, some of the quotes students gave about friends were, 'They hear rumours and make up stories' or 'They know just as much as you do.' On the other hand, of course, the view was that friends are easier to talk to, 'They explain it to you straight in your language'; 'They are on the same wave length'; 'They go through the same things'; 'They have more experience than parents.' This was a recurring theme.

The reason they didn't go to parents was not because the young people had poor relations with their parents, but because they felt their parents were ignorant, didn't know about sexually transmitted diseases, and didn't experience the same kind of things when they were young.

Perhaps youth are right about that. When I was working in an information service myself, parents would come in and look through the books and various resources there. They often chose books suitable for readers years and years younger than their children actually were.

The other side of that is that young people often appear to be protective of their parents in some way, saying, 'Well it is too embarrassing to talk about.' But while sometimes that means embarrassing for the parents, other times it did mean embarrassing for the young people themselves. They were also fearful about parents jumping to conclusions if they asked a question to do with sex. Their parents might think they were having it.

How did young women respond to the information they got from schools?

The school came out as a very very important source of correct information. Wherever a proper health education or human relations program, or whatever it is called, was in operation, in most cases young people were very complimentary, provided the teacher was open to discussion and to questions. They would say very positive things like, 'It's really good' and 'You can go to Miss (or Mister) about anything if you have any questions.' Schools also introduced them to people from other agencies, for example, the Family Planning Association or a community health nurse.

One of the real difficulties young people voiced was that they wouldn't go to the doctor for various reasons. The first one very often was money, 'They charge you twenty bucks.' The second one was, 'It might get back to Mum or Dad.' They are really concerned about the confidentiality of doctors. This was, of course, particularly pronounced in country areas and included the chemist and the welfare centre. Anything in a country town students would just consider off limits, 'Because Mum is a nurse in that place' or 'Our mates work in the chemist and we couldn't go in and ask for condoms.' They would give me the information about which railway stations down the line had condom-vending machines.

Sue, I know this wasn't part of your study, but what are your thoughts about parents who see themselves as the sole source of this information for their children?

I believe that very few parents would consider themselves in that category. Speaking now from my experience as a parent and a teacher, parents who are willing to talk to their children about these areas are usually the ones who don't mind at all if the school does it as well. They encourage the school to do it. It is very often the parent who is afraid to touch upon this whole area who would also be reluctant to have a teacher approach it.

Given that you visited a variety of schools and you also travelled in the country and the metropolitan area, were there any young men or women who were better informed than others?

Yes, in our study we did look at comparisons between males and females and comparisons between metropolitan and non-metropolitan young people. The fact that girls are better informed did not surprise us, but the fact that the country students are so much better informed was a surprising outcome of the study and this goes both for boys and girls.

What do you think that is connected to?

From our data we found that country children seemed to receive more health education in schools so that is obviously one factor. Another reason may be that teachers in country schools know that the children are isolated and so they have a stronger sense of responsibility to introduce this area. Also maybe there is more stability and commitment in country schools as far as teaching staff goes and to become a teacher in the human relationship area you need to build up trust over some years.

Sue, if students are talking to parents, is it both parents?

No, parents means 'Mum' almost entirely. Father is way down the line, after friends. Mother is the first other person students will talk to and some of the comments I got were, 'Mum is always there, Dad is always working' or 'Dad might yell at you, Mum won't get mad.' So students really make value judgements about their parents. Fear that parents may not understand is even more strongly felt in regard to father.

Were there any students requesting information that was in conflict with the values held by their schools or by their parents?

This was a very interesting area. I went to one Jewish school and quite a number of Catholic schools—some co-educational Catholic schools but a number of single-sex Catholic schools as well. In whichever school it was, it came across very clearly that young people feel it is their right to know, and that doesn't mean they will go out and be promiscuous. These are two entirely different things. So they felt that if they couldn't get the information from the school then they were going to get it from somewhere else.

In some cases I challenged them about pre-marital sex by stating that if it was against the Catholic value system to have sex before marriage, and after marriage to have it with one faithful partner only, then sexually transmitted diseases should be of no concern to them. But they got quite hot under the collar and held out that this wasn't the reality anyway, and even if it was, it was still their right to know.

As Kaz Cooke says in her book, 'You never quite know when you are going to bonk.'

Here are a couple of nice statements on that one: 'You need to know to make decisions about your life'—this was from a country Catholic school; and one from an independent metropolitan school, 'You cannot wrap up your daughters in cotton wool and keep them in the bedroom.'

Young people whose parents came from non-English speaking countries seemed to perceive that the background of their parents was different and therefore their morals and their value systems belonged to another time and place. They didn't devalue their parents' value system, they just felt because they were living in twentieth century Australia they needed to know what was going on. For instance, one Catholic girl in a girls high school said, 'You don't want to be scared. You want to know. You need to talk about what you should or shouldn't do. You have got to know or you can't make decisions about your life.'

Sue, what did you find in relation to young women particularly?

I found them concerned about other people and about relationships. I found them very often less embarrassed to talk about these areas than some of the boys.

Was there a discrepancy in the knowledge between young men and young women?

Yes, the young women were certainly better informed. They seemed to take more care in finding out and they had more methods of communication. Girls generally talked to more people about sexual matters than boys did and they seemed to have better sources of information through reading matter such as popular magazines like *Dolly*, for instance.

The boys had nothing to compare with this. It seems that young men are expected to be interested in cars, sports or smutty kinds of sex in *Penthouse*-type magazines. Boys in the interviews felt that there was a gap but they couldn't suggest ways of remedying that. They were very interested in reading *Dolly* or *Cosmopolitan* or some of the other women's magazines but they would not be seen dead buying them. If their sister or mother or somebody else had one of these magazines then they would read them.

Did you gain any idea whether young women are worried about sexually transmitted infections?

Yes, they certainly were concerned about STDs. Of course, AIDS was the big bogey, but I still felt, and this is more a feeling that came out in the interviews, that the whole scenario was not real to them. It was scary, but the issues of relationships, girlfriends and boyfriends, having fun and not becoming pregnant, were more real to them than sexually transmitted diseases and infertility in the future.

Did they know that pelvic inflammatory disease and organisms like chlamydia can cause infertility, and that after one attack there is a 10 per cent chance of becoming infertile, or that after three attacks there is a 75 per cent chance of becoming infertile?

They were almost totally ignorant about this. The best I could glean was that about half or maybe slightly more than that had heard about pelvic inflammatory disease, but their knowledge was very skimpy.

What about Pap smear tests and cervical cell changes or cervical cancer? Did they realise that they should consider having a test if they were sexually active?

Again a fairly large number of girls had heard about Pap smear tests but they weren't quite clear what they were for.

What were young people wanting to know or what didn't they know about contraception?

They didn't ask too many questions on contraception: that wasn't part of the brief. Regarding the consequences of untreated sexually transmitted diseases, I did ask students how they felt about parenthood in the future. I asked them whether they expected to have children once they found a partner they liked and the overwhelming answer was yes. Very few said they didn't want to have children.

The question, 'How would you feel if you couldn't have children?' drew a response of devastation from both sexes. They thought they would feel they were not real men or women if that happened to them. It took away from their gender identity. The group with the strongest reaction were boys of Catholic Southern European descent who said, 'Well, bambinos are part of our extended family and everybody loves children and I love children and this would be really devastating.'

So you didn't get the impression that the idea of women having lives for themselves without children had been considered?

No. They had been thoroughly socialised into believing that children were a normal part of life.

Well there are going to be some shocks for a few of them! Did you get the feeling at any time that you were getting on to taboo subjects?

No, it was more a feeling that they couldn't talk to older people about some of these subjects. They felt they couldn't talk to doctors about concerns to do with sexual behaviour, that doctors were strictly for fixing things up after the event, certainly not to talk to beforehand.

In those schools that had 'good' health and human relations or sex education programs, were there still gaps as far as the students were concerned?

Yes. Perhaps as expected, the best covered areas were changes in puberty—physical changes particularly. The usual plumbing—and the students were absolutely sick of it. The most common complaint was, 'All we get are the basics'. The information was very often unco-ordinated; they would get it in science, home economics and physical education, and it would always be the male and female systems.

The areas which were poorly covered were decision-making skills, values, the consequences of certain behaviour and infertility. I wondered if infertility was of concern to fifteen-year-olds; they are more concerned about not having babies than having them. But there was a really burning, emotional interest in this. Perhaps all the publicity about test-tube babies has alerted them to this.

The lack of communication between schools and medical services in the community was a problem revealed by the study. Students were utterly ignorant of the nearest family planning clinic, of the existence of community health centres or what services they offered. I feel it is really the duty of schools to inform students about available services in the community. There is very good work being done by agencies in these communities, but very often they are not invited into schools. Young people don't know them. Knowing the face of the local community health nurse would do wonders for people feeling threatened about entering this very adult and alien domain.

Community health nurses tell me they are very keen to make contact but of course people can't just enter schools without being invited. Actually, the next stage of our project, had we got further funding, would have been to make these links between schools and community services.

Sue, how do you think young people would like to receive more and better information?

The human factor seems to come up trumps: somebody to talk to, a teacher to talk to, and good discussions in class were highly favoured avenues when it came to topics of personal relevance. Videos were

OK as long as there was a discussion afterwards. Just watching a movie with no discussion about the situation rated lowly, and reading even lower than that. Whatever method was suggested, it had to give young people a chance to put in their own opinion, to talk, ask questions, hear different views, and have the advantage of hearing familiar chatter not only from each other but also from a teacher. Some students said, 'We would like to hear it from a teacher, we would like to hear a teacher use the words about sexuality.' It made it right if they heard the teacher say things about condoms and so on. Then they felt this was something they could talk about as well.

Part III

Bowed But Not Broken

Why is being different a disability?

Fiona Strahan

There are various names for people with my physical difference, such as dwarf, little person, person with short stature or Achondroplastic.

Personally I find 'little person' a bit objectionable. It implies cuteness, sweetness and childlike qualities. 'Achondroplasia' sounds like you're punished for life. You can't go far with a name like that. I mean try spelling it! 'Dwarf' has negative freak connotations too. I tend to say to people, 'I'm short', and take it from there.

When I was young my family and I didn't use any words for my disability. It was difficult to talk about something that wasn't named. When I was born it wasn't clear that something was different so it took some time to diagnose. As far as my parents knew, there was no recent history of this disability in our family.

When I was growing up it would have been helpful to talk about what I was experiencing and what might happen in the future. I had no positive role model to follow. The information I did get was from a 1929 medical textbook. It said I would probably die by the age of 25, with pneumonia, leg and back problems. You can imagine how that scared me. I lived in terror for a while. I built the picture of myself from snippets of information and misinformation.

In one sense I'm glad that my family didn't talk much about my being different or make it into any big deal. I was brought up to be independent, equal and to strive for choice and options in my life. I sometimes think my need to be independent was overdone, because even now I find it hard to accept that I actually need people. The major positive outcome from this goal of independence was in relation to my integration and participation in the community. On the other hand, I've had to deal with a lot of issues on my own and that has been difficult.

I remember when I was about eleven there was a discussion on the radio about using pituitary gland hormones to increase the growth of children who had a particular kind of short stature. My father turned off the radio quickly and nothing was said. So opportunities often weren't taken up to talk about my disability or difference. But in 1959 when I was born, the attitude was that I wouldn't be integrated. Thank goodness my parents had a commitment to send me to regular schools and not isolate me. I think they fought a very unsupported fight in that.

Around this time my father asked me if I'd be happier with other short people. He thought I might be. There is a village on the north coast of New South Wales. I flipped out when this was suggested. I was quite hysterical. I thought they didn't want me.

At school I was accepted for the most part, but there were times when it was hellish. The status quo in peer groups changes so easily. In high school I used to play a lot of sport. I was a really good netballer and a reasonable basketball player. My best mate was joining a team to play in the region, but as I was two inches shorter than the height requirement, I wasn't allowed to participate. My friends and I thought this was unfair and didn't make sense. It was really frustrating. I was equal sometimes but not others.

Even when I was young, before puberty, I felt grown up in a little body. When my breasts started to grow, there were times when my body seemed alien. I was no longer a child but not recognisably adult either. Sometimes when I went to the public swimming pool boys there would make rude remarks about my body.

Once in Year 10 we went on a pub crawl. I met this boy/man who was, I thought, pretty sweet. I was talking to him and he seemed really interested in me and really nice. Then he said, 'I'd like you to come along to my disco because I want you to be the freak show.' I was just devastated because I didn't realise that kind of thing happened anymore. It was shocking. I was unprepared for people to still be like that. There are some really sick people out there.

It was hard when stuff like that happened. I tried to be really brave, really stoic and ignore it. I thought if I reacted, other people would just feel my pain and I didn't want their pity. It's only been in the last ten years that I've actually talked about it in a different way with people, and I've only just started to talk about it with my family.

Another thing that used to happen when I was younger was that people would talk to me as if I had some kind of mental deficiency. I had an extravagant vocabulary then and so I'd give them an extraordinary answer.

I've been incredibly angry with the world and incredibly angry with individuals. I didn't expect people to be nice to me. I believed that my life was going to be difficult. As a woman you work really hard to function in the system anyway. As a disabled woman there are times when I've worked five times harder physically and emotionally. I always feel I'm going to be judged and so I try to interpret what people will think to counteract that. It's like a battle where I have to plan strategies for survival.

I use certain techniques like glaring at people or even sticking my tongue out at them. It's incredibly exhausting. It doesn't create a basis for happiness at all. Yet I need to express my anger. And this isn't acceptable because it's seen as if I haven't come to terms with my disability. But my anger is about not tolerating bullshit. I have to be assertive.

More recently I've had a couple of relationships where I could talk with people and not feel like a freak. They were supportive but not overly protective. Until about eighteen months ago I drank and used drugs to block out the pain. Now I realise I have to let the pain come. I needed to talk about the future and how to deal with people who are rude.

I was really into denial and so were people around me. They would say things like, 'I don't consider you disabled.' And denial is tempting. Disabled is not a nice label when it comes from a society that says I am different rather than saying everyone in society is different.

It's been a process, coming to terms with my body image. I'm lucky that I've always been really outgoing. I've had really great friends. Towards the end of high school we were experimenting with being hippies. We used to swim naked down the local beach and I felt quite comfortable and good about myself.

Then I had an operation. I had some bone taken out of my hip and put in my nose to enable me to breathe better. The doctor said they'd take the bone from behind the hip and that I'd have just a little scar. But they took bone from the front. It was as though he thought, 'Well, in her case it doesn't matter how the scar looks.' I came away feeling totally butchered.

There are a lot of stories I've heard about mistakes in surgery on disabled women and it not mattering; of women going in for one thing and coming out with a numb leg, but because they were in a wheelchair it was as though it wasn't a problem.

At the time of my operation I was just starting my first sexual relationship with a boy. The disfigurement really affected how I felt about my body. Even though I was so different physically, it was the final straw. There were times when I used to say to people that my body was a shell that carried my intellect around. It was like a complete denial of my body as a friend. I've had to do a lot of work in accepting my body. Now I actually like my body. It's not perfect, but it's got some pretty good bits.

That boy I first had sex with bothered to use a condom. I don't think I realised how nice he was until I met other men. When I was young I got a lot of strange messages from my father and also from society that I was asexual and that people wouldn't love me. It took me a while to realise that people might actually want to see my body and that they would like it. After I left school I had a number of sexual relationships with both men and women. I know the outside world was saying things about others exploiting me or, 'Isn't that nice of him to look after her', and not seeing my relationships as a two-way dynamic. My lovers have generally been people who are prepared to look at things and who have a kind of openness.

There are other issues about relationships. Recently my lover and I were walking along the street and this car of yahoos went past and yelled out crude things. Neither of us dealt with it very well. We just ignored it. I can't control that kind of thing, but my reaction was to save the other person, my lover, from it, instead of letting him deal with it in his own way.

I've no idea of what it's like for others to look at me. When I was in America recently visiting my sister, I had my 30th birthday. She asked me what I wanted and I said lingerie. When we went into the shop I wondered if the saleswoman thought, 'What's a person like you doing trying on things like this?' But it was all my own fear and not her actual response at all.

When it came to education, I was discouraged from doing a lot of things. When I was at school I wanted to do drama. A teacher sat down with me and said, 'You can't do drama. You'll never get a decent role.' I was furious but I think he was right. The system out there hadn't changed and wasn't going to in a hurry. That's the hardest thing to accept—the time it takes for things to change. This is what gets me down.

The other thing I wanted to be was a special education teacher. I was told that I couldn't be a teacher because I couldn't use the whole board. So I said, 'That's OK. I'll just rub it out fast.' That was in 1977, a year before the New South Wales Anti-discrimination Act came in. So I thought, 'Well, forget it.'

I've ended up going into social welfare work. I never wrote I had a disability on my job applications. I just fronted up at the interview. But recently, with affirmative action in place, my disability has actually been an advantage. I've been offered jobs that aren't even in the disability area.

I remember someone coming into an organisation where I worked, and where quite a few people with disabilities worked. This person said, 'Oh, so the government's got something for you here. Isn't that nice? Do you get paid? You do? Wow! That's really nice.' We have to put up with idiotic comments like that.

The question society asks is, 'How productive are the disabled? Are they going to be a drain? Will the money come out of our taxes?' Society sees the disabled as being driven around in blue buses with flowers on them. People with disabilities can work. But I also think people have a right not to work.

The state doesn't provide anything for me. For example, I have small feet but don't want to buy kiddy-style shoes. So I have my shoes specially made. I can't claim tax on anything like that. In fact, the state does surprisingly little for disabled people.

Feminist analysis has been of some help, but disabled women have particular issues to address like sterilisation of women with intellectual disabilities. Some women with disabilities in Melbourne have been active in educating the women's movement about their needs and experiences. But the agenda is huge and it burns us out very quickly. Sometimes I am fed up with talking about my disability. There are a lot of other aspects to my life.

I'm fortunate that I'm mobile and economically independent. For some disabled women it take hours just to get up and get dressed or hours to do things in relation to menstruation. So for them it's an effort to participate in activities around rights for the disabled. They think, 'We have enough to cope with. Let people in society make an effort to learn about us.' I can sympathise with that. When I was younger the church wanted me to be held up as a sort of example to others to learn from. I didn't want any part of that.

I share a house with two other women. They aren't disabled. But I have several women friends who are. I tend to make a big effort with women with disabilities. I talk a lot with them and it helps me deal with life, with living. It's too bad that there is so much sexism in the disability rights movement. The men tend to take over. So many women do much of the real work of getting submissions in and getting organisations up but they don't have a high profile in the movement.

Another big issue for disabled women is reproduction. When I was nineteen I got pregnant. That opened up a whole drama because women with disabilities aren't supposed to have babies. We're not even supposed to have lovers. Doctors said things to me like, 'Who do you think you are?' and 'How dare you?' My father said, 'I should have had your tubes tied when you were thirteen.'

But I was prepared to have the baby. In the end I had an abortion. It was decided for me. I didn't really have freedom of choice. It was like short is bad and your child might be short. Disability is bad. You are bad.

About six months after I had the abortion I went into hospital to have an ovarian cyst removed. A doctor who saw me told me that I had no right to have children and I should have my ovaries removed. The surgeon came in later and asked me if this is what I wanted. I started screaming, 'No, no, no!'

I've since had genetic counselling and the message is that my children might inherit my condition. This raises the question about genetic engineering which is of major concern to disabled women as well as feminists. There is a whole concept about eradicating disabilities; people say we must get rid of disability, we must stop it. There's an implication there that people would prefer not to have us around. But we're already here and they can't get rid of us. However, they can prevent others from being born. I don't consider that to be a very nice thing.

I know some people suffer great pain both in a physical and emotional sense because of their disability, but I'd rather see a preventive approach or treatment that would cure or ease their problem. I don't like the word 'eradication'.

I still haven't made up my mind about children. I actually went to the IVF program. They were rubbing their hands with glee when I turned up, because it seemed I was doing the right thing for society. I was looking into having 'perfect' or 'normal' eggs implanted. I had a friend who was prepared to be a donor. I might also look into adopting. I remember a disabled woman who said to me that she wouldn't have a child because society hadn't changed that much. And I thought, society is not going to change unless we lead the way. I won't be satisfied until my situation is not seen as unusual.

Being short is no longer like a ball and chain for me. I am who I am. I'm short. And that's basically all it is. When I see it like that I have enormous freedom.

I never miss it, but yes the earth did move

Mastectomy

Judith Rodriguez

In May 1979 I last saw my friend Emily Hope. She died a few months later, over two years after a recurrence of breast cancer. Hers was the first such illness I'd seen at close quarters.

She had resistance and tenacity which awed me. I admire them even more now that I know I don't possess them—or share them only in a very different form. A jeweller, sculptor and printmaker, she lost the use of her right hand and arm—they were grotesquely swollen with lymph and she carried this terrible burden in a sling. Yet with the left hand she shaped wax on a small length of dowel for casting to make silver rings for a living; and with the left hand she wrote out in exercise books both a journal and the text of the *Legend of Pope Joan*, later published by Sisters Publishing in Melbourne. She also made paintings in tempera and etchings for the book. Even when I last saw her she had a project in mind: an exhibition using many arts and crafts, a shrine to the Goddess.

Emily lived on almost nothing, in sub-standard conditions, in a leaky wooden cottage with an outside dunny. She was not in the same city as her parents. She found it difficult to live with a helper or companion in the house—especially a man she'd allowed to leave his art works in the front room, who came back from a trip and dared to ask her to make him cups of coffee during her working day. (He didn't stay long.) The only thing she would ask me for was occasional help with transport.

During 1979 I reached a decision to leave my husband, and left in January 1980. I had been living in my study in our home, and it was a year of great strain. In 1980 I set up a household for myself and two children. At the end of that year, September, October, I was in Europe, and I remember looking at my breasts in a hotel mirror and thinking, 'That's an odd bumpy bit.'

It had been odd for fifteen years, since I'd had an abscess after my first child was born, which took two incompetent operations and one competent operation to drain. Before operation number one, a medical student had told me that it was cancer, and guaranteed to kill within six weeks. I was distraught—I wanted to see my baby grow older! But the student was wrong, and the result was just a couple of scars and a flattish area above the right nipple.

Fifteen years later, I looked and saw this bumpy bit and couldn't remember what it *should* look like. *My* cancer threat (not really a cancer threat) was a thing of the past but Emily had died. That was enough cancer; surely it was imaginitis, it was on my mind, that was all. Anyway I didn't have time for cancer.

Back in Melbourne some time in the middle of 1981, I began thinking harder—trying to look at my breast one week and the next week, one day and the next day, to compare. But it wasn't until 6 October, when I was at the Bookshelf Gallery opening a posthumous exhibition of Emily's drawings in front of her mother and many friends, that I faced it. In a way, I was facing Emily. The speech I made addressed her directly. It was while speaking that I said to myself, 'This is ridiculous. I'm going to the doctor tomorrow.'

October 7—I made an appointment. October 8—I kept it. The family doctor, my mainstay during unremarkable episodes of bronchitis and asthma, convinced me once and for all by going grey at sight of the breast. Some time before that I'd asked for a complete check-up and he'd shrugged and taken my blood pressure and so on. He'd been my GP during two pregnancies nearly a decade before, he'd often used a chilly stethoscope on my chest and back, but the fading scar near the nipple had never caught his attention.

Next stop: the surgeon, a needle biopsy. Here a very strange thing happened. I had the possibility of being fitted in quickly for the operation. I was resolved on surgery. But I dithered. In some odd way the courteous surgeon made it sound optional: almost certainly cancer—now or in a while—when you've decided. And then, he was up near the Austin, not at the Peter McCallum hospital. I couldn't believe he'd be 'the best'. The sudden perception of a yawning gap in my GP's efficiency had undermined my confidence. So I hesitated and found myself outside, without an operation scheduled.

I got into a panic. I worked myself up to ringing a not-very-close friend, a cancer specialist in Brisbane, who tried to reassure me the surgeon would do a very good operation. But he didn't *know* him.

Then I suddenly realised it had all been left in my hands, and I desperately rang my GP to somehow get me back on the surgeon's schedule. He did, but on 28 October—weeks away.

All this time I was winding up the year's teaching; acting host to a visiting lecturer; doing talks and readings and a review; dining out and going to plays with Tom, who'd flown down from Brisbane;

and taking kids to and from school. I look thin in the photos.

Behind all the activity, and although I was in fact in the fast lane, I considered every hour I didn't get to the operating theatre was a nail in my coffin. By 23 October the surgeon confirmed cancer. I went to see *Amadeus* at the Athenaeum that night, not concentrating too well. On 26 October I had x-rays, a bone-scan in the maw of a huge smooth machine, blood-matching, a cardiograph. Fascinating. I went to hospital. On 28 October I knew as I waited on the trolley that I would have the right breast removed, and a number of lymph nodes which would be examined for cancer.

Now I'm referring to a diary, for clues to my timing motives once I began to suspect I was in trouble.

For the record:

In mid-August I resumed full membership of Medibank—for financial cover, there needed to be some gap between this and the diagnosis of major illness. So—did I delay? I think I did. Was it worth the risk? A year after taking sole financial responsibility for two of my four children, I certainly was not into borrowing, debt, being proved a financial fool. And this was somebody with a good job.

In mid-October came the end of university teaching, before swot-vac. I noted finishing marking tutorial papers. I needed to feel professionally correct, no omissions for mere illness of a kind popularly blamed on stress, 'not coping'.

I did use the diagnosis of cancer as a bludgeon, to hurt. I turned up in the office of the chairman-of-the-year in the English department. He'd tried to obstruct a course I initiated in interdisciplinary studies— even though, being generally against the idea of interdisciplinary studies, he was by the rules of the department not eligible to represent it on the committee in question. I was delighted to pale his face.

Did I use my cancer as a probe? A bit. I hope not. My friends and colleagues were marvellous.

I had to tell my parents. Different reactions, but the saddened look of my father and the visible shock of my mother (safely out of the ten-year check period after throat cancer) both made me equally sorry for their pain. Foreseeing it would be enough to make you delay, I think.

I had no problem about the removal of a breast and the under-arm lymph glands. They'd played me false. Why not the other breast, indeed, if it perhaps was going to do the same. I didn't mind the stitches and scar one bit. (It's been admired by the few professionals who've needed to see it.) I didn't accept suggestions to rub it with Vitamin E cream. My only theory was to live healthily and let the body carry on.

I had little discomfort in hospital. Emily's arm was present in my mind: I satisfied my private feelings by being particularly scrupulous to have my right arm lying level, as advised, or slightly high on a pillow. I did the exercises, just a few times more than they said. Equal mobility of my arms preoccupied me.

I was pretty directly dealt with—just what I wanted. A patch had turned up on the x-ray, in my neck vertebrae. What was it? Either the spread of cancer, or degenerative arthritis. There were more x-rays, and three or four days later he said degenerative arthritis. That was a high. (No arthritic nuisance yet, either, touch wood.) Chances of cancer recurring: six days after the operation I was told— three out of twenty excised lymph-nodes affected, so a 25 per cent chance it *wouldn't* recur. I could live with that (I hoped).

There were several reasons I felt quite good in hospital. I was in a three-bed ward and all the other patients were short-term— elbows, knees, a gall-bladder, an allergy mystery from Mildura. They were very interesting women. Also, as on every other occasion when I've landed in hospital, I found it a blessed relief from petty domestic routine. Yes—full-time cooking and coping and teaching and trying to find time for other things *is* worse than being de-asthma'd in a geriatric ward, though I wouldn't go back for a miscarriage or a long chance on cancer. In 1981 I was judging the *Age* newspaper's Book of the Year award. There were 80 to 90 entries, and they passed from the pile on the left side of the bed to the pile on my right. I was positively blessed with Something To Do.

For days I opened books and read them and wrote down comments, ate good food, fought the noise from the TV room next door, learned to shower one-handed and walked round dangling drainage bottles that clanked. The drainage of lymph had to be allowed to tail off properly—I appreciated this. One day I asked and got permission to go down to the *Age* to sit on the book-judging panel: two small drainage flasks were taped on to my back, under my coat. I went on to drink at The Golden Age with the other judges, and arrived back in the evening, very cheerful, to find parents and children anxiously scouring the corridors for me. They tipped me out rapidly after that: the world was too much with me.

One joyful result of the whole episode was that my divorced husband—the divorce came through while I was in there—who'd said I should never darken the door, etcetera, came with his companion and visited me, invited me to their nearby home to steady me when I got out, and drove me home. It was the beginning of a better relationship around the children.

After all these good things, Tom, now my husband, took me off to the beach with the children. In so many ways, people gave me ease and, though perhaps not in a documentable medical way, an extra chance. They marked my exam papers, brought me bush orchids, wrote me letters, or visited. Wonderful friends.

Chemotherapy: I liked my physician, an odd-mannered but forceful specialist who made off to conferences and who was in the same office building as the surgeon. At the beginning though, going to Brisbane, I had to work hard to persuade him to find me a Brisbane specialist to keep up the chemotherapy routine; he seemed to think I could miss a round of injections! I needed them to keep myself together—they were prescribed, after all. And I was lucky: whether it was my constitution or the dosage, I never felt worse than lack lustre for two days in 28. Blood tests and an injection on the first day; nasty Methotrexate pills on the first day of the first week and the first day of the second week; other pills every day during the fortnight. Then two weeks off, and the cycle repeated. It was to continue for a year, and I was disappointed and apprehensive when the doctor called a halt at seven months. My blood was saying No More.

I refused cosmetic surgery. I just felt like being me, not me-with-attachments. You get used to being lopsided when not in full dress; it doesn't matter.

The prosthesis, the boob: For eighteen months I used the soft little one supplied, and then I bought a good one. It's a nuisance that the brassiere-counter always pretends you need a 'specialist' fitter when buying one. I've always thought it a joke to owe the brand-names and finish of this useful product to its determined other market—drag queens. Jokes about the boob bouncing out when you bend to pick something up, or floating off in the sea, I've never thought very funny. An odd fashion for being 'honest' and going round without a prosthesis I think belongs to angry graceless moments like hacking at my English department colleague. Friends want you to forget, to live forwards—they want to, too.

It's a mixed bag, that On with Life. But things drop away. I used to know the names of all the pills; I can only just recall the feeling of being high and fragile, and mortal, and walking round—in the world, but sharply, clearly separate. When asked in hospital, I didn't want to join a group to go on about boobs, or trauma, or doctors. I offered, later, to go and see women who needed to talk about their cancer, but didn't realise that it's women who are two years past the operation who are asked to do this. In fact I've been able to be useful in this way to one or two good friends, especially round the time of diagnosis and operation.

I regret my lack of kindliness in one direction. Home again, I found myself morbidly 'preparing' my poor children to grow up without me. Even if I'd been about to die within two years, it was hard on them. Maybe I was getting myself an easier life, getting consideration from them, and for that I wouldn't altogether apologise. But the way I thought of it then was as letting them be prepared for anything. Pretty silly: since I was in quite good order, why ruin our time together on a less-than-certainty?

There was a sort of carefulness about physical details after the op. I used to shave under my arms—now I just don't. Don't disturb. Especially after an early episode getting the doctor to drain off lymph that collected in the rib area at the side, under my armpit. ('People will think you just moved the breast along,' I told him.) Being tweaked sharply by the nipple as part of love-making—not now, ever again, and I admit it's out of fear.

Every year since 1985 I've had a check-up at the breast clinic in Sydney, where I've lived a couple of years. Last time all stages of the examination were done by women, which I liked, though I enjoyed knowing my Melbourne surgeon and physician. I don't tell my family when I'm going. It's been nearly eight years. Do I hold my breath? Just a bit—well, you have to, for the x-rays.

During that beach holiday in January 1982, I was being put together again. I knew that Tom didn't give a damn whether I had one breast or two. (I'd have faith in him if it had been a double mastectomy.) I designed three linocuts which I later completed—my first reduction colour-prints. In two of them, I used materials from the Stradbroke Island scrub, and in two of them, the breast and the mastectomy scar were a main part of the design. The first was called Breast and Banksia: the banksia sprig, in black, on the site of the mastectomy, festive as well as death-connected. The second was of twigs, etc. of blackbutt, she-oak and scribbly-gum, with centre-placing given to what I thought of as flayed hide, a piece of bark. The third, Breast Theatre, had a window or rather stage proscenium arch at the site of the breast, opened to show passing clouds and an uprooted, floating tree in colours different from the rest of the print.

Starting a notebook in March, I drew a nice curvy one-breasted nude.

Well, most of that sounds like exorcism, and some of it was innovative and life-invoking. But in the years since, which as it happens have involved moving and halving my earnings, I have also felt tentative about writing and working. I needed the wonderful encouragement when Sisters published a book of my poetry in 1982. The cancer was a stopper, a shock. I looked good to friends but I think I'm still reverberating, I suppose from the cancer episode—or is it moving, or money? And Emily—by my scale of, hold my breath, don't look round, don't overdo—well, what she did with two and a half threatened years was heroic.

I feel a terrible indignation whenever false messages get out about cancer treatment. For instance, when a very sick patient, concentrating on control through meditation and diet, somehow conveys via a bad reporter, or a doctor-hater, to women in an early stage of cancer, the notion that surgery is ineffective—or to be minimised for the sake of a beautiful body—or merely, always, an alternative. Surgery may not be the only answer or it may not be necessary for everyone, but I believe that in my case I am alive because of surgery.

Then there's the distance between private suspicion and diagnosis, the time spent delaying, getting used to fear. How many 'silly' questions or tentative requests for a check-up conceal fear? I think of how difficult it proved to admit to myself that I probably had cancer. I remember how I let pride and fear about money delay facing it. How many women, especially with dependents, 'can't afford cancer'? Or still find they can't talk about it, even now that it's more publicly discussed than ever before? We should remove every deterrent that stops women seeking treatment, both at the first suspicion something's wrong, and later.

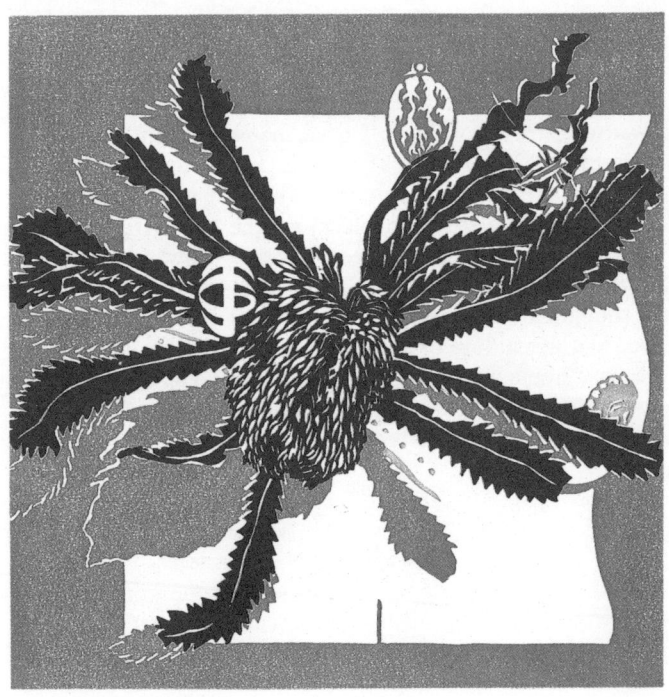

Breast and banksia, Judith Rodriguez, 1982

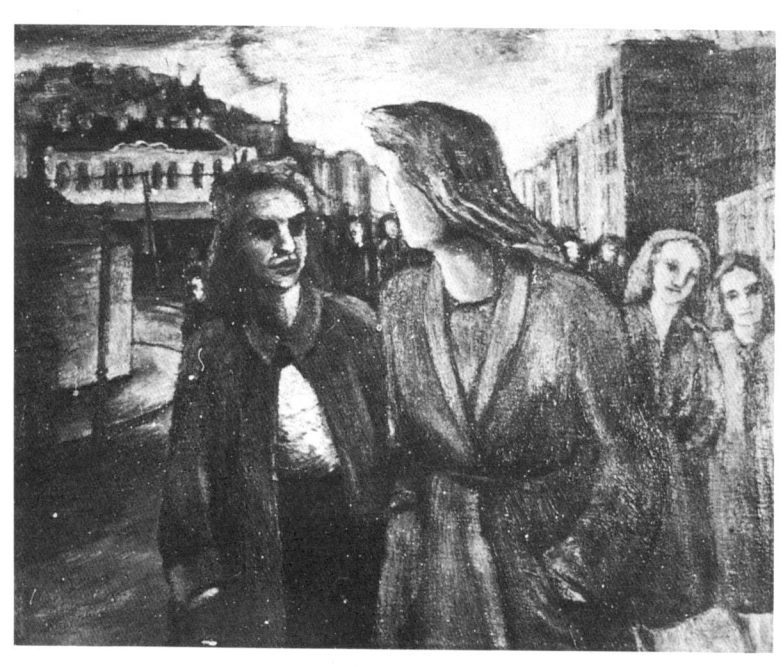

After work, Ailsa O'Connor, 1944

Pride versus prejudice
A lesbian relationship

Lisa Chen interviewed by Kathy Wilson

You are currently in your first lesbian relationship. Can you tell me something about your background?

I was brought up in a very religious family with dogmatic rules about men and women being married and staying married, people always being heterosexual, no homosexual relationships. I was taught those things from a very early age.

And did you believe this yourself?

I thought I did. It is very difficult to tell when you have never been encouraged to question things. That is something I am doing now.

How old are you, and when did you start your relationship?

I am 33. I have been with my lover for almost three years.

Had you previously been in relationships with men?

I was married for nine years. My husband had the same religious background as me. About four years ago, I separated from him. I took my four children and set about creating a new life for myself and them. I remember that leaving my marriage was quite frowned upon by people at church, but I did it anyway.

Did you leave your husband because of your changing sexuality?

No, I don't know if my sexuality was changing at the time. My sanity was. My reasons for leaving were to do with my relationship with my husband. It was pretty bad. I had tried and tried to make it work, following the advice of people at church. But it didn't get better. I was suffering, my kids were suffering. My husband wasn't capable of being a father, a husband, or even of accepting himself as an adult with responsibilities. I left because I wanted a better life. I thought I might, one day, end up with another man who was nicer. But I didn't spend a lot of time looking for someone else. I was mainly trying to get my kids and me settled.

So you were on your own with four kids for a while?

Yes, for more than a year before I met my girlfriend. It was hard going. I was a single mother with four children, surviving on a pension. My ex-husband was harassing me. But being on my own was still actually better than being in an abusive marriage. I felt so relieved.

During that time were you aware of changing?

I was getting a lot stronger but I was still pretty caught up in my family. I spent a lot of time with them. And they were all very religious with a very narrow moral code. In some ways I was changing a lot, and in other ways I was staying the same.

How did you come to start a relationship with a woman? Had you thought about it before?

Never, ever. I met her through a community group that I belonged to. She was one of those people that I liked instantly. I was very curious about her. I used to look forward to spending time with her, although it was always for 'business' reasons. Then I must have started falling in love with her.

What does that mean?

It means I started thinking about her a lot, more than you would just think about somebody that you were making friends with. I made arrangements to see more of her. It was very brave for me to do this because I was a fairly shy person. I certainly wasn't conscious of what it meant. Had it been a man, I would have known.

When did you realise that it was a sexual feeling you had toward your friend?

That is difficult to answer because I never sat down and thought clearly about what was happening. I do remember cuddling with her every now and then when we were saying hello or goodbye. It felt different from how I'd hugged other friends before.

Did your friend know what was happening?

I think so, much more than me. She might have been doing a bit of plotting and scheming. I think she knew that I was attracted to her but that I didn't understand it.

So you became lovers?

Yes, we did. I really revelled in it. I still hadn't given up my religious beliefs but I didn't think about the consequences. I just enjoyed myself.

When people began to criticise me, I couldn't understand why anybody would say it was wrong, when it was such a source of happiness for me. I didn't feel guilty because my relationship with this woman brought me a lot of joy. It was so much healthier than my marriage had been. It was quite ironic that it felt more like the sort of relationship that I had been taught to value and aspire to by the church.

How did you get used to a woman's body after having been with a man? That's quite a radical change.

I was nervous at first. I thought, 'I don't know anything about this.' When you're with anybody new, you're a bit shy and you slowly reveal yourself. But I didn't feel inexperienced for very long. It was easy to admire my female lover's body and to feel passionate about her. That doesn't mean I've stopped liking men per se, or their bodies. I still do.

And what happened with your religious beliefs. Did you just let them fall away?

For a while I kept going to church, thinking that I would practise some of the things that I thought were good, and teach them to my kids. I decided not to decide about the church and God or any of those things until a bit later on. I knew it was too soon, too much for me to work out quickly. It was a lifetime coming to a head.

Did your feelings about your own sexuality change?

The sort of relationship that my lover and I have made together means that I am much more in touch with my own feelings, which also means my sexual feelings. I'm much more of a sexual being than I thought I was before. I've surprised myself.

How did your family, friends and kids adjust to your lesbian relationship?

I hadn't told people about my relationship with my lover, so to them she was my new friend. We spent a lot of time together and my family resented that. My kids liked her. They were making friends.

Then my ex-husband found out. He had a dream about me being

in a lesbian relationship. During our marriage he had often flown into huge, probably even clinically mad, rages and his dream triggered him off. I remember he came to my home, violent and abusive. It was frightening. He swung from moralising to uncontrolled cursing and swearing. I still have an image of his face, his eyes swollen with anger. And that was the beginning of the trouble.

He started involving members of my family in what he thought was his job of 'cleaning everything up for the children'. He and people in my family had a lot to say about what I could and could not do. He threatened to take the children away from me and at one point he did that. He abducted the children. He didn't see it as abduction, but that's what it was. It's interesting that he did it on the day our divorce came through. I think he never truly believed that I would go through with the divorce. My lesbian relationship was an excuse used for venting his fury at me for leaving him. It gave him opportunity not motive.

I had to initiate proceedings in the Family Court to get the children back. What happened in court was horrifying. The outcome was that my children would only be returned if I undertook not to expose them to my lover at all. My barrister told me that if I didn't do this, I would be unlikely to get my children back.

My ex-husband recruited some of the members of my family to say that I wasn't a good mother to the kids, that I didn't care for them, and wasn't looking after them properly. He told my family that I was in a lesbian relationship.

Why was it that your family could be recruited to speak against you?

Because of the religious aspect of it. They were highly outraged that I was in a homosexual relationship. I think that my actions also meant that they'd each have to ask questions about themselves, in order to accept me. They saw me as 'evil' and believed I had to be punished.

Did you make the undertaking?

I was forced into making it. I don't see it in any other way. I knew it was a terrible position to be placed in. It was so awful I almost didn't believe it could happen.

In the court proceedings was your sexuality raised as an issue?

Yes it was raised as an issue and it was absolutely unjust. The court became the forum where my ex-husband could try to humiliate me. And that was more of what I had been fighting against in my marriage. The undertaking was an incredibly inhumane thing to propose, and it came from him, through his barrister. I felt assaulted that day, and it was called 'for the welfare of the children'. It was like the court became another of his weapons. They asked me to choose between my lover and my children and at the same time, made accusations about me not caring about the kids, not being a good mother and even not wanting them. They were asking me to prove these things by choosing my lover rather than my children. Of course, I chose the kids because there was no way I could let them go. It truly was a question of their welfare and it was the only way I could prove that I was a 'good' mother, that I did care. The choice wasn't reasonable—it wasn't a choice. Either way I lost—and that was how our arguments had always been.

What happened with your lover?

She stuck by me. She was hurt and angry too, but she stayed. I remember she said, 'If our relationship is going to break down it will be because of us, not them.' She was very strong and clear. She supported me the whole way through all of this. I don't know how I could have done it without her.

Did that mean you had to organise times to see her when the children weren't around?

Yes, it was very difficult. I was suddenly on my own again with the kids. They were in strife. I had little money and no babysitters. My family had helped out before. Now they wouldn't and my lover couldn't pop in, smiling, being with me and talking to the kids. There were no more outings. But we did it. We had a love affair by late night telephone. Occasionally I could visit her at work during the day. Also, my husband had weekend access so the kids were with him some of the time.

You mentioned that at one point your husband actually abducted the children. What happened?

He kept them for a week and a half. They ranged in age from three years old to nine then. The youngest one hadn't ever been away from me before for that amount of time. She was very distressed. She didn't understand and I don't think anybody explained it to her. All the kids were in a mess by the time they came back.

They'd been told a lot of terrible things about me. My ex-husband didn't have any reservations about calling me a whore, a sinner, a slut . . . He said anything he could think of to destroy the kids' trust in me. He really tried to convince them that I didn't love them, didn't care about them, and didn't want to be their mother anymore. It worked, although less so with the younger children.

The two younger kids are girls, the two older kids are boys. For years the boys, especially, had been craving their father's love. Even though the girls had some of the same feelings, they were probably a little more attached to me. So it was harder for my ex-husband to break that attachment. When they came back my sons were very angry towards me. They had problems left over from when we had lived with their father—maybe I contributed to them. I remember telling them to love their Dad and to keep on trying with him. (That's what I was doing and believed to be right.) I may even have given them the message that added to their vulnerability to him.

Before the abduction and the court proceedings my lover and I and the kids had all been having a pretty nice time together, gradually making friends and getting used to each other. One night Sam, my oldest boy, came into the loungeroom after waking up and found me and my lover kissing. I probably looked pretty shocked but he just said, 'Oh don't worry mum, it's not the end of the world,' and went out again. I thought it was a really nice thing to say.

But when Sam came back from being with his father for that time he was very different—hostile, antagonistic and seeing me as an enemy, not his mother anymore. My sons had been told that because I was with a woman it meant that I no longer loved them because they were male. I didn't realise at the time how deeply worrying this was for them. It didn't even cross my mind, probably because it was so untrue.

Your children had been asked by their father to choose?

They may have been told it was a choice, but in fact it was no choice. They were worked on. It was a really terrible thing to do to them. The information he gave them was so distorted. It played on their fears.

Every time the kids came back from visiting their father they were very distressed. The older ones were aggressive. The younger ones woke up crying in the middle of the night and looked pretty dazed during the day, obviously not knowing how to deal with their feelings. On most access weekends my ex-husband made terrible scenes at the front door screaming abuse and threatening me. Once he came back with the children, returned the three younger ones and said, 'Come on Sam, let's go,' and took him back to his house.

This was even though the courts had given you interim custody of the kids and you had undertaken not to be with your lover?

Yes. I didn't know what to do. Sam was saying that he didn't want to live with me, that he wanted to be with his father, because his father was the only person who really cared about him. That outraged me. It was such a lie. This man had done hardly anything toward looking after any of the children. I didn't know how to tell Sam that he was being deceived and used. It was so sad. I felt so desperate and furious.

Then he talked my second son, Richard, into going too. He used the same promises and the same lies. Richard had been missing Sam, that was extra leverage. I haven't succeeded in getting either of them back. My ex-husband continued to enlist the help of some members of my family. The court counsellor, who knew I was in a lesbian relationship, was very biased in favour of my husband. She believed everything he said and nothing that I said. That was very difficult, because in the Family Court system a court counsellor's report is almost gospel.

Even though I fought the court counsellor, my family and my ex-husband, I still lost two of my kids.

They've damaged my kids a real lot. I don't know if Sam and Richard will ever be able to realise who I really am and disbelieve the lies they've been told about me. I don't know if I'll ever be able to recover the relationships I had with them, and they were good relationships. But they couldn't withstand the force of the things being done to them, and I couldn't help them.

Did you have any help as you were going along?

Yes. My lover helped me. She kept me sane through the worst parts. I also had help from a family therapist. She encouraged me to keep on fighting. She was very supportive and sensible. She saw the prejudice in my ex-husband and family and how they called upon that prejudice in other people. My solicitor was also incredibly good.

It would have been a long haul?

Nearly two years. I don't know how my lover managed to stay with me. She's a very strong person. But I know she felt guilty, perhaps more than me. I refused to say, 'It's all because of us that the boys are gone.' It was people's reaction to our relationship and their hostility.

How have these experiences affected your relationship?

It's stronger in a lot of ways, scarred in a lot of ways. We are still recovering from those years we spent trying to save the kids, and trying to keep everybody sane. We're very tired. And that makes me sad. It's really cost me a lot personally, but I wouldn't have done anything differently.

Have you resolved issues about who you are, and being in a relationship with a woman? Is it comfortable for you?

Very, very comfortable. Yes I have resolved it. I plan to be doing it for the rest of my life. I want to stay with her for a long time. She's very nice.

But you still have the loss of your sons to deal with?

Yes. And in a way my girlfriend has too. She sees me struggling and hurting. She's done a lot of work with my daughters. There's often a lot of sad and angry feelings around. Life is hard some days.

Is your relationship healing after the unsatisfying relationship you had with your ex-husband?

That's a hard question. Forgetting whether she's a man or a woman, I picked a very good person this time. She happens to be a woman. I get a lot of pleasure from her womanliness.

Are you living with her now?

Yes, with my two girls and her daughter. We make a nice little family. We work to make it satisfying. I think that is necessary for any family. Families aren't magically terrific.

And how do the kids cope with living with two women who are lovers?

They cope very well with it. I don't know what they will do if they get flack from kids at school, or other people in their lives. So far, they enjoy being with us and being a part of this family we have created. Our daughters are OK.

At school, we've been accepted very well. They are friendly to us, and supportive of our kids. They treat us as they do other members of the school community, which is very good. We've had mixed reaction from our friends. Some of our friends have disowned us completely, and others love us as usual.

Has your family ever accepted the situation?

No, not at all. My mother keeps saying she has a psychologically damaged daughter.

Are there any other things you would like to say about yourself and your life now?

Well, yes. Five years ago, I don't think I could have imagined myself being where I am and doing what I'm doing today. At the same time, I'm not surprised. In some ways I've changed a lot, but I'm not really a different person. I feel better as a person. And that's a lot to do with the fact that I'm in a good relationship. It's not to do with whether my partner is male or female. It's to do with the fact that my partner brings out the best in me.

You smile as you say that.

Yes. My relationship with this woman of mine makes me smile and feel happy. Our sex life is very good. It's not shocking at all. Gosh, why did I say that?

I think there are people who have accepted the idea of homosexuality, and I think there is another group who are horrified by it. To that group I want to say that homosexuality is not a horrible thing. For me it has been a very good experience and still is.

Beyond wifedom and motherhood

Mary Mahoney

When you marry and have six children you lose a bit of who you really are and become primarily somebody's wife and somebody's mother. There was a time when I thought that identity was really important, but then I had to start finding out who else I might be. It's been a long journey.

I have been married for 22 years. When I got married it was the done thing. If you didn't have a boyfriend by the time you were eighteen or nineteen you were on the shelf, like this was a serious problem. It's probably similar now.

I never questioned whether that was what I wanted to do or not. I just accepted that that's what women did. So I met somebody, and started going out and it got serious and I remember feeling safe. I thought, 'I've now got a boyfriend and he wants to marry me, and things are going OK.' So we decided to get married. But when I look back, it was decision by indecision. I can't remember sitting down and thinking, 'This is the rest of my life I'm talking about. Is this the person I want to spend it with?' We just drifted into getting married.

But I was probably a little unconventional even then. I didn't want to have the big white wedding, although I was pressured into it by friends and by my mother. A lot of people look back on their wedding day and say it was wonderful. I hated mine, being the centre of attention and dressed up in this stupid, fancy dress. I felt silly.

After we married, I started taking the pill. I didn't know anything about it. Because I was a Catholic, I went through all this mental trauma, but in the end I took it, even though I felt guilty. It affected my body very badly and I often felt sick. It was awful, so I went off it and became pregnant straight away. This was nine months after I married.

My husband and I had never actually sat down and talked about having children, how many we wanted or who would mind them.

It was just assumed that I would have babies and look after them. I fell into the role—I became a wife so easily, it frightens me. I changed from an individual who was involved in the Labor Party and anti-Vietnam marches to this docile little wife. I actually used to get up and cook my husband's breakfast every morning before he went to work!

It was after I had my second child that I read *The Female Eunuch* by Germaine Greer, which had just come out. It really got me thinking and it changed my life. She was out here, on telly a lot, promoting the book. It was all really big news and I loved her. I thought she was a great woman. I started questioning the fact that I was doing housework and child care round the clock every day of the week. I talked it over with my husband and negotiated some time off for myself.

Reading Germaine Greer was the first spark in my awareness of women's issues, but I had a long way to go. I still craved more children. It was really an addiction, now that I think about it, but at the time I thought of myself as an earth mother. Physically I gave birth fairly easily. I felt strong and could really celebrate my body. I continued to have children. With the first four I really liked being pregnant and the births went smoothly. I loved breastfeeding.

When my fourth child was about three I wanted another baby, after all, it was something I could do well and feel good about. I had some difficulty conceiving this time and when Jamie was about four I remember thinking, 'Jamie's going to be at school next year. If I don't have a child at home what am I going to do? I don't have any excuse for staying home, either. Who am I?' It was a feeling of panic.

But then my body came to the party and I became pregnant again. I was thrilled. It turned out I was carrying twins and this time it wasn't a good pregnancy, revolting in fact. I was quite sick the whole time. I was 34 and it took a toll on my body.

When the twins were born, I breastfed both of them for eighteen months! I was exhausted and not coping very well. I cried a lot. I had too much to do and not enough time to do it. I'd been keeping active in the Labor Party and I'd set up a women's co-op. I've always had to do things outside of the home, to keep my sanity.

But I felt like my life was falling apart. I remember feeding the twins one morning. There was cereal from one end of the kitchen to the other, and both had dirtied their nappies. I went out to the laundry. I used to wash them in this big sink and change them on top of the washing machine. I remember being out there and my husband coming out to say goodbye, because he was going to work. I said, 'I can't do it.' He asked, 'What can't you do?' I said, 'Today

I can't clean up the shit, and the cereal and change their clothes. I can't do it.' I burst into this heap of tears and ran upstairs, leaving him in his suit to clean up all the mess.

It was a turning point for me. That's when I really started to read and think a lot about my life. I remember times when people would ask, 'Do you work?' And I had always said, 'No.' But I started thinking, 'If I don't work, then how come I'm so bloody exhausted all the time?' So I began saying 'Yes, I do work but I don't get paid for it'—all sorts of things to raise awareness for other people but also to help me describe what it was I was doing. I started questioning every aspect of my life and that was increasingly hard on my relationship with my husband. My mother died about that time, too, so you see, everything was up for grabs.

Money was also an issue for me. My husband earned a good income and he never told me how to spend money or held any back. But I never felt it was mine. I felt guilty if I bought something for myself instead of for the children. In our society, like it or not, money is an important way of feeling good about yourself. My self-esteem was way down, rock bottom, because I felt that I had given up a lot. I was a good student at school and wanted to go to university. But I left school in Year 11 because we had no money. I can remember my father saying to me, 'Why don't you go and get yourself a job, and buy yourself some nice clothes?' When you're seventeen it sounds like a great idea. I worked in a bank and then I worked in an insurance company. I actually did a job that I quite liked.

But I got married, had six kids and became financially dependent on my husband. I didn't know at the time how much I would regret not having any qualifications, qualifications that count anyway, and how important it would become for me to be financially independent. One of the things that traps women is their financial dependence. In recent years I've had this great sense of wanting to be free— free to do things for myself without thinking, 'Who will mind the kids? Who's going to cook the tea?' The constant responsibility is a huge burden and one which women carry often without even questioning.

I had been totally conditioned by my Catholic upbringing that a woman's duty was to raise children, devote herself to them and that it was the best thing a woman could do. I think it's a lie. Mothers are treated like dirt. We are never made to feel we are doing an important job. Society's idea of rewarding mothers is to send them a flowery, sentimental card on Mother's Day. It's unbelievably superficial and the rest of the year, who cares?

As a Catholic I was also taught that a mother is the best person to bring up her children. Then I started to realise that the issue of child care was absolutely crucial for women and that we had to stop thinking and perpetuating the myth, that the only person who can look after a child is its mother.

There are a whole load of options for caring for our children that the community has to take responsibility for. Everyone wants you to have a baby and says how wonderful it is, but they lock you in a house in suburbia and leave you to it. So there are structural, societal and political aspects to the issue of child care. The personal is political, as the women's movement says. Why should men be free to participate fully in society and women restricted?

The capitalist system needs women locked up in little suburban houses, freeing the men to do what they do. It all props up the system. It's dangerous to do things differently and to think differently about ways of caring for our children. It's dangerous to allow women to participate fully in the system. I mean, things might change!

There is some talk now about child care for women in the paid workforce which is good and needs to be acted on. But we shouldn't forget that a woman at home needs child care too. In 1980 I got involved with some other women in setting up an occasional child-care centre in our local community. We set it up as a women's co-operative and it's still going strong. We need to provide options for women, not just rely on grandmothers and other women friends to help out with child care. That's women again taking it on.

The centre allowed women to have space from their children without the need for excuses like, 'I have a doctor's appointment' or whatever. Why couldn't they just leave the kids and go for a walk along the beach, read a book or have a rest—all those 'self-indulgent' things that women aren't allowed to do? We encouraged the women to leave their children without a word about why they were leaving them.

I also saw how unhappy so many women were from staying at home all the time. They were talking about their husbands in such derogatory terms. They felt they had no control over their lives. I identified with that. My husband could ring up at six o'clock and say, 'I'm in a meeting and I'll be home at half past seven or eight o'clock.' And I had to wear it. What can you do? You've got six kids at home. They've got to be fed. I would have loved to be able to just ring up and say, 'I'm not coming home till eight o'clock.' But I couldn't do it.

And it is so boring being at home all the time. I mean really boring! There is nothing mentally stimulating about it. Yet I get furious when I hear people saying how dull housewives are because all they talk about is their kids and making sandwiches at the canteen. But what else can they do?

As well as the child-care centre, I became involved with Action for World Development (AWD), which is where I work now three days a week. I met and began talking with other feminists, and that was very important.

As I mentioned before, I was questioning all aspects of my life. I looked at women's position in Catholicism and at the age of 38 I actually left the church. I did it very formally. I wrote a letter. It was an important step for me.

I questioned the role of sex in my marriage. I always slept in the same bed as my husband, but there was a period of three months when I was celibate. I told my husband I needed to sort out whether I was having sex because I wanted to or because it was my duty as a wife and my husband needed it. Was I feeling guilty if I said no?

Also there was the thing about affection and sex. If I showed any affection at all my husband would think I wanted sex. A lot of men respond emotionally only in two ways—either with anger or in a sexual manner. I know women who are afraid to smile at their husbands because they interpret it sexually! I made a decision that I would not have sex if I didn't feel like it, and I've stuck to that.

I talked it over with my husband. I told him that when I say no I mean it. And I explained that it has nothing to do with not loving him or being angry at him. He handled it well. I know other men who call their wives frigid old cows if they don't want sex all the time. One of my friends is going to a sex counsellor for this reason. It's very important for women to start defining sexuality for ourselves and not just in men's terms.

Another issue that came up was the issue of women propping men up, protecting them from facing reality sometimes. We've all got them sitting on our shoulders. I decided this wasn't on if I was going to be true to myself. My husband would have to start dealing with his own stuff. He didn't take this very seriously at first, but now he's joined a men's group, and funnily enough is finding it very rewarding relating to men on a more intimate level! I believe this will be a very important model for my sons.

I've tried to raise the issues concerning women's roles with my daughter and five sons. But I recognise that, for the boys, my husband is their role model, not me. And I know that society demands a certain amount of conformity to what is considered 'masculine'. I can't change my family overnight.

But my children certainly know what the issues are for women. When one of my sons was in Grade 6 he was the only kid in the class who knew the word sexism in relation to advertising. My oldest son is living with a woman friend now and they share the housework, and are trying to do things differently.

Our routine at home is also shared now that I work outside of the house and the kids are older. Three kids each cook tea on the three days I work. I actually only cook twice a week. My husband cooks once a week. We buy a meal one night and that's been good. He and I share the washing. The kids take total responsibility for their own rooms. I've relaxed my standards a little too. My kids go out with scruffy shoes or with holes in their jeans which is the fashion now and I've had to accept that. I know one of my kids smokes marijuana and that's OK. I've encouraged my children to be independent and tell me straight out what they want. I may not always agree, but we can negotiate.

I've struggled hard to get my life in shape and I'm really looking forward to the future. I think I'm finally starting to feel a bit freer and in control. That can only be good for all the people around me. I feel much better about myself. I'm really excited about where I am now and what the future holds.

Part IV

Back to Basics

Wisewoman or witch
The herbal tradition

Sue Evans and Assunta Hunter

We live in a culture in which, for the last few thousand years, there has been an imbalance of power between the sexes in favour of men. This has been going on for so long that it takes some effort to really register its implications.

Take a moment to imagine how it would feel to live in a society where the situation was reversed: where 95 per cent of the world's resources were owned and controlled by women; where positions of power and importance in business, government, the arts and education were filled by women; where the pronoun 'she' was used to refer to both female and male; and where the female human body was accepted as the norm and male bodies were described only inasmuch as they differed from female ones. How would it feel to be a woman then?

Medicine, we know, invariably reflects the culture from which it develops. Western medicine, like all our sciences, can be described as extremely rational and masculine—left brain, if you like. It emphasises cure rather than prevention, and dramatic intervention in the disease process rather than a reliance on the inherent self-healing capacities of the body. Because most of us have never experienced any other type of medicine, it does not occur to us to question its most basic principles.

Once again, let's imagine. This time, imagine there are ways of treating illness that redress imbalances, rather than treat specific disease states. Imagine ways that look at promotion of health rather than elimination of disease, and that use medicines with long practical application rather than ones based on recent scientific research and quantified clinical results.

Those who have had experience of natural therapies will recognise these characteristics as typical of that form of medicine. It may not be so widely known that traditional medical systems such as Ayurveda (from India), Unani (from the Arab States) and traditional Chinese share a similar focus.

In the West, medicine is defined as 'what doctors do'—a very narrow definition. Doctors do, of course, practise medicine, but they are not the only ones who do so. We kiss a crying child's bumped knee and (s)he immediately returns to play. A friend or neighbour, feeling lousy, drops in for a chat and leaves an hour later, feeling much better.

These are everyday experiences and, we would argue, medical ones. The distance between these and the sophistication of organ transplants and microsurgery may seem light-years, but both are effective in alleviating human suffering, though not used interchangeably. It is as potentially disastrous to try to talk someone through acute kidney failure as it is inappropriate to give painkillers to a child when a kiss will do.

Herbalism has long been the traditional medicine of women healers the world over. And like the role of the healer itself, herbs and how they have been perceived in different cultures at different times can be a useful reflector of socio-political change. Gone are the days when both women as priestesses and herbs as their tools were revered. Now, in many 'modern' cultures, herbs are regarded as second-rate medicine and women as second-rate citizens.

In ancient shamanistic cultures, the rituals of life were conducted by and for women, as much as men. And their tools were the herbs which linked them with the power of the land. In these societies, healing was a divine art and the priestesses were as powerfully connected with the earth as their male counterparts. Their status was equal to that of the priests, but there was recognition of their unique role as women. The old religions paid homage to the Mother Goddess as the birthgiver who ushers life into existence; and to man as the Horned God, the hunter, the one who faces death.

Even today, in hunter/gatherer societies, the collection and preparation of herbs as medicines is an extension of the woman's role as the major food provider. Their knowledge of plants and their habitats and seasons, as well as their uses, has always been a special aspect of female learning. The wisewoman in these cultures is always one who knows much of herb lore, whatever else her ritual and social wisdom may be.

It was in the second and third centuries before Christ that male supremacy in both religion and healing began to exert itself. In Egypt, women were no longer seen among the deities or their earthly representatives, the priests. And the kinds of healing open to women— domestic and women centred—were gradually accorded a lower and lower status. Women continued to practise, of course, but their kind of healing no longer had the authority of religion or the status of the public world of male medicine.

By the time of ancient Greece and Rome there was another aspect of social change which further downgraded women as healers. It was the growth of formal education and universities. Formal knowledge began to be valued over the practically based experience which had always been woman's domain. As the centuries rolled on, this rift became still more polarised as the gap between science and superstition. By the twelfth and thirteenth centuries, long after Christianity was established in Europe, the persecution of herbalists, midwives and wisewomen shows the extent to which society no longer valued women. The devaluing of herbal medicine took some centuries longer, but it was part of the same gestalt which lost sight of the traditional wisdom and status of women.

Aesclepias, one of the earliest healers in Greek mythology, is credited as saying: 'First, the word; second, the plant; third, the knife.' We may adapt this to: 'First, the word (or talking through); second, the plant (including diet, plant remedies and other natural therapies); third, synthetic pharmaceuticals, and lastly, surgery.'

The political implications of diagnosis and treatment are very real. Using herbs as medicine is a political act which can link us to an ancient tradition which is in the true sense 'popular' medicine. It is the medicine of the people. Tending a herb garden, or making chamomile tea to encourage sleep in a restless child, or making an ointment from marigolds to help heal a nasty rash is a way of healing we can all use.

As the nurturers of children and the food preparers, women have maintained an understanding of the place of herbs as special foods. Healing the family is a vital, if often unacknowledged, aspect of female wisdom. Those who developed more sophisticated skills, for example, the herbalists and midwives, often paid dearly for their trouble. Is there a relationship between the lack of European herbs which are documented as being useful for women's reproductive problems and the witch hunts? Is it that there are really so few suitable European plants compared to the North American tradition, where there are so many? A more plausible explanation may involve the frequency with which herbalist midwives were accused and convicted of witchcraft. It is likely that in over four centuries of burnings, much valuable knowledge was lost.

Of the knowledge that has remained, here are six plants which have a broad range of uses, many of which relate to specifically female ailments.

Chinese Angelica (Dong Quai)

This strong and upright plant may sometimes grow to ten or twelve metres, with an upthrust umbrella of seed pods. It is the Chinese and Indian varieties which have such a well-deserved reputation as friend to the female. They are valued in the East as plants which help to regulate the female reproductive system and restore the female body after both childbirth and menstruation.

The angelica has a broad range of uses, since it balances, feeds and cleanses the system. It can ease menstrual cramps and irregularity, as well as many pre-mentrual symptoms such as headache, irritability and fluid retention. As a hormonal balancer it is also useful at menopause or after childbirth. It should not be used in pregnancy or where the menstrual flow is already excessively heavy. The dried root can be bought through any Chinese herbalist.

Nettle (Stinging Nettle)

This is the nettle which stung so fiercely when you were a child. It grows in many vacant blocks and all chicken coops. As with many of the useful and safe plants of the world, the nettle can be a food as much as a medicine. It contains useful amounts of iron, vitamin C and chlorophyll, and cooked as a green tastes like sweet spinach.

Like angelica, it is a tonic which strengthens and supports many systems in the body. It can be used to relieve excessive bleeding and haemorrhage and, of course, helps to replace the iron lost. It is a gentle herb that we often recommend as a tea for pregnant women. It combines a mild diuretic action with an iron supplement: a handy combination in pregnancy.

German Chamomile

Here is a herb familar to many of us as a night-time tea to help us sleep. It has many other uses also. Most centre around its mild, soothing properties for nervous tension and related disorders such as digestive irritability and gastritis. It relaxes the nervous system and acts as an anti-inflammatory.

Marigold

Common marigolds (Calendula) are widely grown in public parks and private gardens. Their cheerful orange-coloured flowers bloom for many months of the year and they self-seed easily.

One of the most interesting uses of calendula is in the treatment of painful menstruation. It has a reputation for regulating periods when they are irregular, and moderating excessive menstrual bleeding. As it has an oestrogenic action, it is also useful in menopausal difficulties.

Chasteberry Tree

This small tree is an attractive Mediterranean plant with lovely purple flowers in late summer. It likes lots of sun. The leaves are pleasantly aromatic, but the part used is the berry.

Like many of the herbs we use, its precise mechanism of action is unknown. It is believed that, in some way, the herb influences the pituitary gland, enabling the production of oestrogen and progesterone to be balanced.

Chasteberry is slightly progesteronal, making it a favourite with sufferers of pre-menstrual tension. Remedies like chasteberry work by stimulating the body's own regulatory processes, in this case, balancing the production of hormones.

However, hormonal imbalances which lead to such distressing complaints as PMT (pre-menstrual tension) are not always due to excessive production. They can also be seen as a problem of excretion, leading to a build-up within the system. The liver plays a major role in the elimination of hormones from the body. Here, naturopathic treatment would involve the use of such liver herbs as dandelion and bayberry bark, with chasteberry playing a more minor part.

The rebalancing of hormonal production post-pill is another situation where chasteberry is valuable. The suppression of ovulation which makes the pill such an effective contraceptive can cause problems when a woman wishes to re-establish her cycle, often when she wishes to conceive. Chasteberry, again usually in combination with other herbs, is frequently prescribed by herbalists in this situation.

Arrach

This is a little-known plant which grows in Australia as well as in its native Europe. Culpepper, writing in the 1600s, is generous in his praise for its actions on the reproductive system generally: 'I commend it for a universal remedy for the womb, and such a medicine as will easily, speedily and safely cure any disease thereof . . . '

As we must always remember, herbs do not work on specific conditions, for, in themselves, herbs do not heal. They provide the conditions within which the body can heal itself. It is only shorthand to say, for example, 'This herb is good for painful menstruation.' What is meant is that a particular herb has been found useful in allowing the body to heal itself.

Arrach has recently found a place in the treatment of endometriosis. Other symptoms reported to be eased by arrach include PMT, menstrual clotting and painful periods.

Conclusion

All these herbs have a long history of use, either domestically or within more formal healing traditions. Many have fallen into disuse in recent centuries and we wonder what other herbal treasures are awaiting rediscovery.

As history is rewritten to include the experience of women and to revalue their lives, we will reconnect with many of the understandings of the Old Religion. We personally feel a responsibility to continue the tradition that, according to some estimates, eight million women died for in the European witch hunts, between the fourteenth and seventeenth centuries.

Within our lifetime we trust that the word 'witch' will lose its association with evil and once again become synonymous with wise woman.

The husband even thanks the butcher

Nutrition in a social context

Pat Crotty interviewed by Rose Sorger

Pat, why have some aspects of nutrition and health been given attention over others?

Various things influence which nutrition problems people worry about, or which issues get on to the agenda for public discussion. Coronary heart disease, for example, is a major concern, and one which I think comes from a medical orientation to food, eating and health.

Do you think doctors have had more to say about nutrition than social scientists?

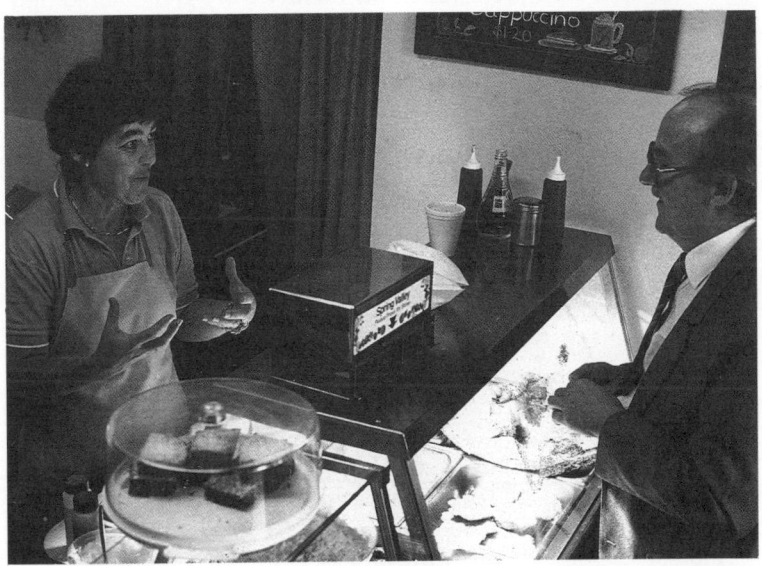

Woman in food shop, Joyce Agee, 1989

More than their share, I think. Social science is at a disadvantage, because medical science tells people they'll die if they don't change their behaviour. It's the ultimate threat. Social scientists take a different approach. They ask questions about people's needs or motivations and try to understand what's going on, whereas medical scientists usually try to understand, and teach other people what they understand, and what they think should be done to change a particular undesirable situation.

Why don't people look to social scientists for this information?

When it comes to being objective, medical and natural scientists hold the high moral ground in deciding what is fact and what is not. I think a lot of people in medicine see social science as 'mickey mouse'. It's more complex, less black and white, and it certainly doesn't have the status of medicine.

Women have traditionally had a lot of power and control in relation to buying and preparing food. Is this still the case?

Yes, but in a way women's responsibility for buying and preparing food in the home is a double bind. Firstly it demands a lot of their time, because families have high expectations of women in this role. At the same time, 'deskilling' of women in relation to food has also occurred. Take food preservation for example. My grandmother, my mother, and maybe yours too, used to make jam, used to know about fruit and its seasons. Women today have lost most of that knowledge and expertise because they don't need to use it anymore. You can buy jam and other ready-prepared stuff now. It's much cheaper in terms of time, which is the valuable commodity now. Thus it's an interesting paradox that food can be both a source of power for women in families yet a disadvantage to them too.

Women who are tied to the traditional model of household duties buy, prepare, present and clear away food. How difficult is it to challenge this model?

There's been an important change in family life in Australia over the last decade and more women now have not only domestic responsibilities but an outside job as well. In families people are bargaining to do fewer chores, at the same time as women are trying to share the load. Usually it still falls on the woman. Negotiating family tasks is an area where there's a lot of pressure.

Another example of this difficulty is when women are trying to lose weight. They often say that it's a problem if they have to handle food, and they'd prefer not to. When the kids ask for biscuits, it's hard for them not to want biscuits too. This issue is not strictly a nutritional one, but it makes the point that when we educate to change what people eat or how they eat, these issues have to be considered too.

Is there a potential for conflict if women really want to change those roles?

Not for all women. For example, I live by myself and I do whatever I please, but for most women it's a delicate balance. Dale Spender has written about women's role in keeping the peace, and how it is never counted as work, although it's so difficult and demands enormous skills.

In some families changing roles works quite well, but in others it is tremendously difficult. In households from cultures where the male role is dominant and women are seen as servants attending the family, it certainly has a potential for conflict.

What other lifestyle changes have affected the way people eat?

There has been a shift away from families eating together. People tend to eat out more often now, at different times and places—although some still keep up traditional meals, like lunch together on a Sunday. Children and young people are now more independent—they buy their lunch at school, or at a shop, or they're old enough to eat outside the home with their friends, in fast-food restaurants.

Do you see any similarities between education about diet and food, and sex education?

Yes, and I think that's because nutrition education, sex education, and religious education too, are similar in that they are all highly moral areas. Most people fairly easily understand that religious education and sex education are based very much on values, which means a wide range of views can be presented, but I'm not sure they see nutrition in the same way.

Although a lot of advice about food seems objective, this is misleading because it's very much to do with values. It has a moral background, so to speak. For example, in health education, women who are overweight are sometimes judged as 'letting themselves go'. Food is linked with over-indulgence and that's seen as bad, while abstemiousness is seen as good.

It's really hard to separate a fact from an interpretation of the meaning of that fact. Sometimes in debates about food, people become intensely passionate about an issue, believing they have the facts; whereas in truth their argument is based on one of an enormous number of possible ways of interpreting the facts.

Do you think that people who are interested in making a profit out of weight-loss programs have tapped into women's anxieties?

I don't know what the turnover is in the weight-loss industry, but it's likely to be enormous if you include syndicated weight-loss programs like Weight Watchers and Jenny Craig—special dietary products, the huge range of off-the-shelf products and the equipment that goes with keeping fit. Then there's the clothing industry, which is built around the image of having a thinner, athletic, leaner looking body. So, how women look is an important cultural theme for business and commerce.

It is sometimes very difficult to sort out a humane non-judgemental way of dealing with variations in body shape because people in our society have negative reactions, particularly to a large female figure. In an interesting study GPs were asked about unpopular patients. Although alcoholics were at the top of the list, overweight people came either second or third in terms of their unpopularity with doctors.

Women who asked questions were probably unpopular too!

And if you're overweight *and* ask questions, you're really in trouble!

A lot of this is happening at a subliminal level, isn't it?

Yes. The messages about women's shape often come across in a fairly subtle way. For example, it may be just the kinds of women we see on the TV screen, and thus the kinds we don't see. Maybe ten years ago, I remember somebody saying to me, 'The only overweight women you see on TV are behind bars, in *Prisoner*'. It was hard to think of anybody who was overweight in a good role.

Despite all this, if you are overweight it's not all bleakness and no quality of life. In one study, women were asked about their satisfaction with their body shape and their relationships, and a significant group of overweight women were satisfied and happy. So it's obviously possible to feel OK about yourself and the world and your relationships, even if you don't conform.

Pat, there seems to be a vacuum in regard to nutritional information about things like calcium supplements. The dairy food industry, or pharmaceutical companies who manufacture vitamins, often step into this vacuum and tell women they need six glasses of milk a day or a certain number of supplements. What do you think about this?

I think the whole area of nutrition information is just fascinating, particularly because it is so persuasive in nature. As for vitamins, this is one of the major areas of change in nutrition as far as scientific information goes. Fifty years ago we didn't even know of the existence of all the vitamins, whereas now you can buy them in health food stores in unlimited quantities. We really don't know the implications of that.

It certainly could be true that women in particular are subject to persuasive messages about food and nutrition, and that's an area which hasn't been studied enough. There's so much information, it can become very confusing and there are few guidelines to help people find their way through the maze.

Not only the commercial sector puts out these messages either. Various agencies like the National Heart Foundation, the Anti-Cancer Council, health departments and other public or independent health organisations are constantly multiplying and churning out messages about food.

I would like to see people have a more sceptical viewpoint about nutrition, because it's not only the Australian Meat and Livestock Corporation and the Dairy Board and so on who have vested interests. The National Heart Foundation and other health groups have them too. They want people to behave in a certain way, because their mission is to persuade people to eat less fat, or whatever. However legitimate that might be, it is very confusing to hear all those messages.

We need to help people develop the skills to sort out for themselves the useful and relevant information they need to solve their particular problem.

Another issue for women is that many of the messages about diet are often exploitative, and this includes those from legitimate health educators. 'You should do this for your family' can play on women's guilt. They feel guilty even if this is not deliberately intended because of the way women are brought up in our society. For example, many women whose husbands have heart attacks feel guilt that they might have caused the attack because they used to give him fried fish. He liked fried fish and they were never game to argue with him, so they assume the guilt. I don't think we've addressed those issues at all.

The best way to educate people about diet is to strengthen their confidence in selecting information for their own needs. That involves rejecting information from any source when they don't need it or it doesn't suit them—maybe even from a legitimate health education group. If we did that, our health education would be quite different.

Can you imagine women forming nutritional groups in their own communities?

Certainly I can. Currently in the United States local community nutrition councils are having a lot of influence. Similar small groups here could work with local councils or district health councils. There's a lot more opportunity to address local concerns about diet in that way than if a program is centrally organised.

It would mean a broader range of issues could be considered, not just coronary heart disease. It might include homeless kids, because they often have nutrition needs and problems that make eating very haphazard, or the elderly might feature as a priority, or maternal and child health might come back into fashion. When people talk about coronary heart disease, my reaction is always to wonder about health issues for old people and mothers and babies because somehow they've been forgotten.

With local groups there'd be a lot more motivation for people to get involved. It wouldn't be someone 'up there' telling them they should eat low-fat foods. It would be more flexible, they could go ahead and develop their own recipes or ways of cooking that would suit their own lifestyle, whether they were young people sharing a house, or a traditional family. If you're skilled and confident about it, you can take the message and make it your own.

A question for some women might be how to manage when it's the end of the social security fortnight and they only have five dollars to spend.

My guess is that different women use different skills to tackle this problem. We might think that people with less educational experience will be less able, but I question this. Maybe not everyone with only five dollars can do well, but some people can do very well. For example, this time when the money's running low you might call in your favours from friends you have helped in the past when they were in need. There might be some kind of networking arrangement so that your kids go over to their place for tea those two nights. These are the areas that social scientists and workers in nutrition and health are interested in.

Has there been much money put into research of these important nutritional areas?

This is close to my heart, Rose. In the past, nutrition research has been largely along medical lines, which means it's been about disease and food-choice relationships. Just now, a group of us has received funding to do a study which will involve both traditional nutrition techniques and more qualitative information. It will seek out information not only about what people's actual diets are, but also about their problems and how they deal with those problems. It will sort out the skills they use, the strategies they put into practice. We were surprised to get the money—grateful too—but surprised because of the tradition of medical emphasis in funding nutrition research.

So I hope that this will be a boost for people who work at the practical level of service in the community—an opportunity to gain information from a study which will be practically useful for them. They might draw people together then, to share those strategies. I'm sure they'll be the sorts of things that a dietitian like me would never think up. I could probably recite to you the general thinking about preparing budget meals, but that's often not very practical because it's born out of technical knowledge, and not out of the need to know what works, what's practical.

What can we celebrate about women and food?

There are lots of things to celebrate because food has been our business for so long. In hunter–gatherer or other tribal societies, about 80 per cent of all the food was gathered by women. It might be more stunning for the men to come in with a kangaroo that they'd killed, but that only happened once every few days, whereas all along the line women kept things going. That's an image of women as quiet achievers—they've always been in there with their skills. Maybe that hasn't been recognised enough and maybe it can be exploited. You prepare for a family, what do you think?

Well, I think it's an area of great satisfaction for many women, but you need time and money to be able to purchase the food. It's often very creative. You have a spirit of being generous to other people, but I'd agree with you that it's also open to exploitation especially when people just sit down and eat after taking no part in the preparation or in the cleaning up process. Children often choose not to see what is being done, or will not take up the skills. One's always fighting sexism in the kitchen.

Maybe meals should be more of a big deal rather than just routine. The fact that we have them three times a day means we take them for granted. Maybe we need a bit of PR on the family to show the importance and the difficulty of the work with food.

If a woman withdraws her labour, which I've done, that can show how much it means to people. It's seen as a great loss and provides an opportunity to review the situation and people's role in it.

There's a lot to do in family settings in order to change those values about meal preparation. In some television advertisements for food, meal preparation, and the women's role in that, is seen as trivial. They say things like, 'It's so simple if you use our particular brand, just heat it up and put it on the table.'

Or they make it seem that, after all, the butcher's the one who's done the work, because he's cut it up into those little 'instant' pieces!

And the husband even thanks the butcher, doesn't he?

Country Practice

Roslyn Bayliss

I am 33 years old and the mother of two girls, one nine and the other almost three. I am a doctor, and for the last six years I have been the only general practitioner in a country town in Victoria, several hundred kilometres from Melbourne, and 300 kilometres from Adelaide. The nearest base hospital and specialists are at a largish town over 100 kilometres away.

In many ways our town could be considered a 'typical' small country town. The shire has a population of 2000 people, 900 of whom live in the township. It is predominantly wheat and wool country, and in the past has been quite prosperous, although the last few years have brought hardship to many. There is a secondary college providing education to Victorian Certificate of Education level. The town has a ten-bed hospital and a nursing home of similar size. The hospital is not permitted to provide obstetric services. There is a voluntary ambulance service.

My practice sees about 150 patients per week, including hospital and nursing home patients. I am on call whenever I'm in town—which is most of the time! There is, of course, 'no opposition' as such, although some patients prefer a doctor who is older, or male, and travel 40 kilometres to the next town. I receive about the same number of patients from that town, who come to me because they prefer a doctor who is younger, or female.

The same problems come up again and again. Some I know are specifically 'rural' problems, others I'm not sure of, and some others are problems faced by women everywhere. What I propose to do is to introduce you to some of the women who have come into my surgery over the past six years. Through their stories I hope that you will come to understand the problems they face.

The people most likely to be aware of the disadvantages of rural communities are the 'itinerants': people who have moved to the town, usually from the city. These people include teachers, bank staff, professional people and women who have married 'locals'. These people bring with them certain assumptions and perceptions that need to be reassessed when faced with the realities of living in a small country town. This compromise can often be quite difficult.

Wendy came to see me some months after moving here from Melbourne. She was pregnant with her first child. She had worked with children who were brain injured during birth, and she was scared about her own delivery.

Being from the city, she was used to the idea of specialist obstetricians in big teaching hospitals being the norm, and was dismayed to discover that the nearest obstetrician was over 100 kilometres away. She knew no one there she could stay with, and the thought of driving that distance while in labour was a frightening one.

Her fears were increased when she learnt that the hospital here was not able to provide obstetric facilities, and that the baby would have to be born in one of the nearest towns, 40 kilometres away. I assured her of the skill and care of the doctors in those towns, of the excellent safety record for mothers and babies attended by GPs in small country hospitals, and the relatively low rate of intervention as compared with the larger hospitals. Being small does have some advantages. She left my surgery reasonably reassured.

In the event, all did go well. But it is hard for women who come from the city, where there are obstetricians a short drive away, and a plethora of doctors and midwives to choose from, to change their perceptions.

As you will see, isolation and lack of choice are the root causes of most problems faced by rural people. A good example of this is the problems faced by those women who come to me wanting an abortion.

The demand for abortion is probably about the same as in the city. However, the difficulties faced by the person requesting it are quite different. Two women who have approached me recently for a termination illustrate these difficulties well. The first was a 40-year-old mother of four. She and her husband were struggling to make ends meet, and the prospect of another child was, to say the least, a daunting one.

The other was a sixteen-year-old girl. She had strictly religious parents who had forbidden her to see her boyfriend. Unfortunately, she had no independent means of income, and no transport.

For both these women, each quite different, the need for an abortion posed the same problems. The first hurdle was to tell me. As the only doctor in the town, they had no other choice as a source of referral, yet they have to play badminton with me and attend the same parties. Many of my patients find this awkward. These women were no exception. Then they had to find an excuse to go to the city for a couple of days, and find the means of transport to get there. These factors combined to turn what would be a stressful experience for anyone into a time of real difficulty.

Naturally enough, people in the country, as in the city, hold differing views about such emotive issues as abortion. Unlike the city, however, in certain circumstances these issues can split a rural community in a very public way. Several years before we came here, the high school attempted to introduce a compulsory sex-education component into the curriculum. This very quickly became the subject of heated and acrimonious debate. In the end the idea was shelved.

A couple of years later, the same subject was offered as a non-compulsory unit, under the name of 'Health and Human Relations' (I am often invited to be a guest speaker at these classes). There has been no controversy over this at all. I am unsure whether this reflects changes to the attitudes of the community, or the cleverness of the school's curriculum committee!

Being a mother of preschool-age children is another stressful experience that living in the country can exacerbate to almost intolerable levels at times.

Kathy brought her six-month-old baby to see me on a few occasions because he was crying so frequently. After much listening, examining and discussion we agreed that he was a normal, healthy baby. The real problem was Kathy's stress.

She lives on a property about 50 kilometres from town. She moved here from the city when she married a farmer, leaving her family, friends and full-time job as a teacher. Before she had a chance to return to teaching locally, and thereby make people's acquaintance, she became pregnant. She is now alone with her baby for at least twelve hours every day, seven days a week.

Kathy's husband keeps promising that it won't be long until his workload eases and he can spend more time with them, but there seems to be a never-ending stream of problems for him in managing their new property during a particularly unkind year.

Kathy comes into town two mornings each week, but she doesn't know anyone that she can either leave the baby with for an hour or two, or even just visit herself. She would be more than happy to pay someone to babysit, but who? There is no family day care or child-care centre that she can avail herself of. Her frustration is mounting and unless I can help her find an outlet, there'll be an explosion in herself, or in her life.

However, it is not only child-care for babies that is lacking, but the whole spectrum of child-care facilities: parental relief for an over-active toddler or preschooler, after-school and holiday care for school-age children with both parents working, school-time care for a sick child of a working mother, daytime care for a preschooler with a working mother.

One of the hindrances to the development of child-care facilities is the widespread notion of, 'You bore the children, so you should care for them'. This is perpetrated by community groups, grand-parents, relatives, husbands and, most frustrating of all, by a large proportion of the mothers themselves. These mothers see preschool child-care as a luxury, something which they even feel a little guilty utilising, and until this attitude is changed, child-care will never receive the priority it needs.

For women like Kathy, who need child-care facilities for their own well-being, the guilt is magnified, because they see this need as a product of their own failure as a mother.

It is difficult for those women who work, too, because there is widespread community disapproval of working mothers. Some em-ployers in the town dismiss women when they marry or reach 21. My friend Sandra, mother of three primary school children and full-time high school teacher, confided to me recently that she felt sick with dread if one of her children complained of feeling a bit off-colour on a school night. Who on earth could she get to care for them if they were sick the next day?

The opposition these working women face from other women annoys me because farmers' wives work. They do the farm books; they cook and rouseabout during shearing; they drive trucks and tractors during harvest; they feed the dogs and chooks. But many refuse to see this work as anything other than an extension of their housewife duties.

Sandra and Kathy are by no means atypical. Time and time again I see women in my surgery who present with stress-related illness caused by problems with their children. I consider the provision of adequate child-care to be a pressing health-care issue in our town.

I do not seem to attract the same criticism as other working mothers, probably due to the high status still accorded the medical profession in rural communities. I have noticed, however, that any behavioural problems that my children exhibit are instantly blamed on difficulties they are presumed to experience because I work.

Lack of public bus or train transportation in our town is another problem. This means people without cars can't get access to health services in larger centres. It also affects the elderly. Agnes is 92 years old, and fit and healthy. She's also lonely. She is a widow, lives alone in her own home, and doesn't drive a car. Despite having lovely helpful neighbours and friends, despite actively attending Senior Citizen's Club, church meetings, and Day Centre, she is still stuck with long, lonely evenings. She would love to call on her friend Edna who is in exactly the same position, but there is no taxi to call and she feels that she already makes too many demands on her friends for transport. From time to time she has a 'holiday' in hospital, and absolutely thrives on the company.

Things were even more difficult for Annie. She was 94 years old when I first met her. She had always enjoyed excellent health and had never before consulted a doctor. She told me that she didn't believe in them.

Her husband had died twenty years earlier and three of her four children had moved away. She lived alone in a huge sandstone house and her meals were delivered from the local pub. Until recently she had continued to drive out to the family farm once or twice a week. This had changed when, for good safety reasons, her licence was taken from her. This broke her heart, as she became totally dependent upon the goodwill of neighbours and friends, and she was left with no opportunity for independent movement.

I was asked to see her because of hip pain due to osteoarthritis. This condition meant that any extended walking was out of the question. Had she lived in a larger town, she could have used a taxi service to get around (she was quite wealthy enough); even bus travel would probably have been feasible. As it was, however, she was trapped in her house, and her health started to deteriorate, more from frustration than anything else, and she had to move into the nursing home.

The breakdown in family and community networks in the country has been delayed compared with the city, but nevertheless it is now occurring at an ever-increasing pace. While I am aware of the negative aspects of this strong family network, it also offered many benefits to those supported by its nurturing web. Those extended family/ community support structures are not being replaced by welfare-type structures.

Local community members are trying desperately to take up the broken threads left by the breakdown of the extended family. There are a lot of voluntary groups and services evolving. Let me give you a few examples.

A couple of young women were struggling with the problem of obesity and wondered how best to help themselves and others in this position. This has developed into a self-help group called 'The Achievers' Club', which deals with all aspects of self-esteem, fitness and appearance, not just weight. There is a weekly get-together with such activities as aerobics, swimming, demonstrations on make-up and clothing, lectures and videos on various health topics. The members phone up one another during the rest of the week if they are feeling depressed, or are tempted to overeat (the two seem frequently to go hand in hand). Almost incidentally, many kilograms have been shed in a sensible, healthy and inexpensive way.

The local group of the Nursing Mothers' Association of Australia is a very active, effective one. The numbers at the meetings are usually about fifteen or twenty, and the discussion is comfortable and open.

Sporting activities such as tennis, aerobics and squash are the main leisure activities for women. They provide the opportunity for social interaction, respite from children (co-operative child-care is either arranged formally or occurs spontaneously) and relief from stress, as well as physical fitness, all of which are basic for the maintenance of good health.

I find practising in a rural area to be a richly rewarding experience. It is true that I miss the support of peers. Continuing education is difficult, as is trying to provide objective medical advice to people I have become close friends with. But my work is always varied, the people friendly, and the country is a great place to bring up children.

Somtimes Mum gets
called for advice or
to come over to people's
places I get rathersad that
she gets so tired

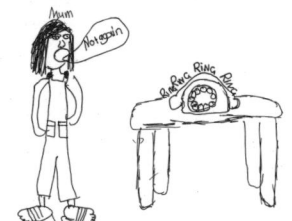

On the way to footy we have
to stop at the hospital.

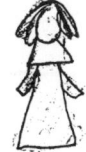

Drawings by Seren Trump, daughter of Roslyn Bayliss

Part V

Low Ebb

Women's despair, women's lot?

A feminist overview of depression

Margaret Goding and Linsey Howie

I had various levels of depression over the years. Probably the worst one was where I was actually deluded into thinking that people were going to come and take my children away because I was an unworthy mother . . . I felt filthy. I had tremendous guilt and remorse. I used to lie in bed at all hours of the day, which was ironical because when I went to bed I couldn't sleep anyhow, and if I did sleep I used to wake up in anxiety. I was very, very flat. I couldn't talk to anyone very much. It was a great strain on my resources just to deal with my family . . . I didn't bother to bathe myself . . . I didn't clean the house. I didn't do any washing. I didn't cook meals . . . If I did get out of the house, it was a plodding wander around the place. There were all sorts of symptoms but those were the worst, and again this dreadful fear pervaded the situation. I just had this shocking fear that I was out of control.

(Reproduced with permission from *Ecstasy and Agony*, forthcoming publication by D. Grounds and J. Armstrong.)

Being born a woman in Western society makes it very likely that at some time in our lives, we will feel depressed. Women are treated more often for psychiatric illness by general medical practitioners than men, and are more likely to be prescribed mood-altering drugs than males. In Victoria, for example, an analysis of community surveys carried out by Ellen Berah showed that more than twice as many women as men were diagnosed as depressed. Some argue that it only appears that women are more often depressed than men, because they are more likely to disclose how they feel emotionally and are more likely to seek medical help. But the responses of the sexes in community surveys which include those who have not sought medical help show that the differences are real, not an artefact of differing 'illness behaviour'.

Origins and causes of depressions

Some researchers claim mood changes depend on fluctuations in hormonal levels. Because women experience the regular hormonal changes of the menstrual cycle, and more dramatic changes occurring with pregnancy, childbirth, breastfeeding and menopause, their state of mind reflects the state of their hormones.

But there does not appear to be sufficient evidence to view hormonal changes as a major cause of depression in women. All women who give birth experience a dramatic drop in progesterone levels, yet only some women are diagnosed as clinically depressed after childbirth. Women appear to be in a vulnerable state, as evidenced by the third or fourth day 'blues' that most women describe, and this may be related to hormonal factors as well as to the major adjustment of becoming a mother.

Menopausal women do not necessarily become depressed. Emotional difficulties appear to be more often related to role transition issues of children leaving home, or perceived loss of physical attractiveness. Hormone replacement therapy, although in many cases alleviating physical symptoms, does not appear to have any long-term effect on emotional adjustment. We could regard hormonal changes as bringing about an increased vulnerability to depression, rather than simply as a causative factor.

Bonding and loss: According to psychoanalytic theory, early satisfactory bonding with the primary object of love, usually the mother, is the basis of self-esteem and well-being in later life. The early loss of the loved person, whether by death, lengthy or permanent separation, or serious neglect, can lead to vulnerability to loss and depression in later life. But this theory does not explain why women are more at risk of depression than men.

Female psychology and socialisation: Some believe that women are more vulnerable to loss of relationships because relationships occupy such a central place in our lives. Feminist therapists Susie Orbach and Luise Eichenbaum see this propensity to form and value relationships as a result of female socialisation. Girls are brought up to prize relationships with loved ones and to gain the greatest rewards from the approval of others, so that they experience greater loss of well-being and self-esteem when that relationship or approval is interrupted or lost. Boys, in contrast, are brought up to be more independent of others, and so are less susceptible.

In psychoanalytic terms, depression is viewed as anger turned against the self. When we link this to our understanding of female sex roles, we can see that because it is not acceptable in our society for girls to be angry or aggressive, anger may more often be turned inwards in this way, and lead to depression.

Sex-role stereotyping: Depression has been described (by Ryan) as a 'very typically female form of distress in the sense that it is a passive and socially inoffensive mode of being . . . It exudes power-lessness and it is the antithesis of activity and control.'

We cannot underestimate the power of cultural mores in shaping individual personalities. From birth, children learn behaviour and ways of thinking which are seen to be appropriate to their sex. Girls learn to be passive, dependent on others for direction and satisfaction, to take pride in their physical appearance, and to nurture and look after others. They learn to be helpless as they cannot control what is happening around them.

It may be that being 'good females' in our society predisposes us to being depressed. In one landmark study in the United States, Inge Brovermann and her colleagues asked mental health clinicians to use a list of personality characteristics to describe the 'mature, healthy, socially competent woman' the 'mature, healthy, socially competent man' and the 'mature, healthy, socially competent adult'. The 'healthy female' was frequently rated as more submissive, more emotional, more easily influenced, less independent, less competitive, and more conceited about appearance than the 'healthy adult' or the 'healthy male'.

It seems a powerful negative assessment of women existed. More-over, while the profile of the healthy male was almost identical with the profile of the healthy adult, the profile of the healthy woman was markedly different. The implications for women are serious: either they can opt for the healthy male/adult role, take on more 'masculine' characteristics and be regarded as socially unacceptable because they are not 'womanly'; or they can try to conform to the 'feminine' role and be more prone to depression, since research by Tinsley and others indicates that women who fit the traditional model of femininity are more likely to become depressed than other women.

Are women's lives depressing?

While the theories examined so far go some way to explaining why so many women become depressed, it is only considering the social hardships facing so many women that enables us to recognise that the causes of depression are not simply a matter of individual pathology or predisposition to illness.

Women and work: Women earn less than men for various reasons. They are more likely to be unemployed, especially young women.

In addition, many women with children either work part-time, or move in and out of the workforce, or leave paid work for some years, all of which lowers their incomes. Overall, women in paid work earn on average only 69 per cent of male earnings. But even when they work full-time, women earn only 80 per cent of average male full-time weekly earnings (1988 figures), partly because typically 'female' occupations tend to be lower status, lower paid occupations such as sales, clerical work and service.

Women and social security: Nearly two-thirds of pensioners and beneficiaries are women. More than 80 per cent of single parents with dependent children receiving social security are women. These women are in a poverty trap, often lacking job skills, access to education or adequate child care, and facing financial disincentives to train or enter the workforce. This trend is called the feminisation of poverty.

Women in the home: A Victorian Ministerial review into Education for Health Promotion in 1984 identified women with three children under fourteen in the home as a high-risk group for depression. Other high-risk groups were the unemployed, the recently bereaved and disaster victims. The susceptibility of women in the home to depression may well be linked to various aspects of their situation: the long hours of unpaid work, the low status, the isolation and the lack of alternatives, such as child care or opportunities for paid work.

Older women at home who are responsible for aged or disabled relatives are another group for whom recent research indicates high risks of depression.

Women in danger: Forty per cent of homicide victims are female, while women commit less than 5 per cent of all murders. Assault in the home and sexual assault are also overwhelmingly committed by men with women as victims. The Victorian government's inquiry into community violence was presented with strong evidence on increased incidence of depression experienced by women following sexual assault.

A social understanding of women's depression: After examining the above ideas and data, we endorse the view of George Brown and Tirril Harris that depression is essentially caused by social conditions. In a survey of 500 London women, they found that working-class women were four times more likely to be depressed than middle-class women.

In their analysis of the many factors involved, they found that difficult life events or ongoing difficulties precede the onset of depression in women, but only when other predisposing factors are present: lack of an intimate confiding relationship; having three or more children under fourteen at home; not being in paid work; or losing one's mother before the age of eleven. Working-class women are likely to have more of these factors operating more intensely over longer periods of time.

These external factors cause the woman to construct her internal personal world in a way that manifests in her becoming depressed. Depression is the price she pays for adaptation to her perceived social reality.

Dealing with depression

In traditional psychiatric medicine, health professionals are taught to classify mental illness or disorders according to the American Psychiatric Association's *Diagnostic and Statistical Manual of Mental Disorders (DSM3)*. Depression is considered under the heading of 'mood disorders', and mood is defined as a 'prolonged emotion that colors the whole psychic life' and generally 'involves either depression or elation'.

Depression is discussed in terms of degrees along a continuum ranging from depression as a natural human emotion including sadness, dejection and disappointment to severe depression where delusions may be present and where suicide is a risk.

Symptoms are described as psychological or physical. Psychological symptoms include depressed mood with accompanying gloominess, sadness and dejection, a sense of hopelessness and despondency, feelings of worthlessness and guilt, difficulty in thinking or concentrating and indecisiveness. Loss of appetite and/or loss of weight may be present along with insomnia, whether it is difficulty getting to sleep, or waking through the night or early in the morning.

When women are depressed they may experience a sense of either agitation or slowing down or both. They may also experience a generalised anxiety, lowered self-esteem, feelings of inadequacy and diminished sexual interest. Some women feel better in the evening than in the morning. Physiological symptoms may range from headaches, dizziness, heart palpitations and cramps to nausea, indigestion, vomiting and constipation.

It is worth commenting at this point on what we might call the 'medicalisation of melancholy': that feeling depressed, which in many instances can be seen as a natural human response to loss and powerlessness, has somehow been taken over by the medical profession. Many women, wondering whether their distress is real, or whether they are 'overreacting' seek reassurance from medical professionals. These 'experts'—mainly men—sit in judgement dispensing treatments that respond to *their* perception of what is 'normal' often not taking into account the reality of women's lives.

Most women with depression do not need to be hospitalised. However, when women become severely depressed, hospitalisation either on a voluntary basis or on the recommendation of two doctors usually occurs. In hospital, women will receive medication or electroconvulsive treatment (ECT), and some form of therapy, whether individual, group and/or occupational therapy.

A standard approach to dealing with depression includes anti-depressant drugs, sedatives and anti-anxiety agents and neuroleptics for the treatment of agitated depression. Anti-depressant drugs relieve depression by elevating a person's mood. The most commonly used are the tricyclic anti-depressants—amitriptyline, protriptyline, nortriptyline and impiramine. Some brand names include Tryptanol, Concordin, Nortab and Tofranil.

For women to have a feeling of control, it is important that they be informed about anti-depressant drugs. For example, they should be told that it may take a week or more before an elevation of mood is experienced. Possible side effects can include a dry mouth, blurred vision, constipation, drowsiness and lowered blood pressure which may result in dizziness. Ways to counteract some of these problems (for example, acid sweets or gum for dry mouth, fluids for constipation) are outlined in publications such as McSwiggan and Sweet's manual for nurses.

Some women may become dependent psychologically and physiologically on anti-depressant medications and they need to be withdrawn very carefully and slowly from them. Unfortunately, many women are prescribed medication for many years without adequate review or consultation, and sometimes without any recommendations of alternatives such as self-help groups.

Also, while we know that serious depression always carries the risk of suicide if left untreated, anti-depressants may not necessarily avert this risk. If a woman is deeply depressed and is given anti-depressants, there is some risk that, as her depression lifts, she will become active enough to kill herself, and may hoard the pills as a means of doing it. Close monitoring is thus necessary.

Electroconvulsive therapy (ECT) consists of passing an electric current through the brain. For some severely depressed women, it has been effective in alleviating their depression. But short-term, or even permanent, memory loss is a common side-effect. Also, for some women, it is frightening and disorienting, involving an extreme sense of loss of control. Since loss of control over one's life is often a major contributing factor to depression, we can hardly see ECT as a long-term solution.

While some women express favourable outcomes post-ECT, and we do not wish to diminish their relief or sense of well-being, we believe it is a controversial treatment that should be used sparingly and with the utmost care and sensitivity.

We have stressed the limitations and problems of hospitalisation, medication and ECT, how they often deal only with the symptoms rather than provide a long-term solution. Yet in some cases their temporary use may be vital in ensuring that a woman remains alive.

Feminist therapy

In recent years feminist writers, such as Anne Edwards in Melbourne, have made a significant contribution to our understanding of gender bias in theories about mental health: the extent to which therapists hold different standards of mental health for their male and female clients; the tendency to over-medicate female clients; and the reluctance of health professionals to consider the influence of social and environmental stresses and gender-role stereotyping in shaping women's lives and compounding their distress.

Knowing what is considered mainstream or orthodox psychiatric practice in our society empowers us to challenge conventional wisdom and to find or create alternatives that reflect women's experiences and meet women's needs.

Medication and ECT are not solutions to a depressing life of economic and social hardship. They do not change the understanding of the woman by enabling her to take charge of her life and raise her self-esteem. They do not change the functioning of her family (except that the family and society now label her as 'sick in the head') and they do not change the structures of society. They are individual, not collective, approaches.

In medical terms, depression comes to be viewed as undesirable. Although we know that depression is not a pleasant experience, exploring this 'dark side' may open up new and creative possibilities. We must trust our own feelings and allow the free expression of grief, sorrow, despair or anger.

As feminist therapists, we explore the contexts of women's lives—how women have incorporated the damaging messages of sex-role stereotyping into their everyday existence—and we challenge social adaptation that is at the cost of women's health. We believe that the best therapy for depressed women happens with a therapist who is female and a feminist.

The first task of the therapist is to be supportive and nurturing towards the woman and accepting of her misery. Together, the woman and her therapist develop a clear picture of her context, including how she grew up; important relationships, past and present; social networks; economic and working conditions; self-nurturing, if any; nutrition and exercise; and past attempts at dealing with depression.

The therapist needs to convey to the woman that her hopelessness is a reasonable response to her life conditions, not some alien state that has descended upon her. The process of therapy will involve reframing the woman's experience in a way that makes sense of her depression and avoids shame and guilt.

Past and current losses must be recognised and grieved for; often women who are depressed find it difficult to cry deeply with full release. Being given permission to cry in the presence of an accepting person is healing.

Learning about anger and how to express it safely, how to ask for what you want, how to be proud of what you can do, and how to apologise less, are behaviours that women can begin to practise. They need reassurance that they are not thereby betraying the older generation of mothers and grandmothers, who clung to traditional 'feminine' ways as their only means of survival. Women need to understand that they will not fix themselves by trying harder to be a 'nicer' person, and that giving up 'nice girl' behaviour will not be easy. The therapist and client can work together to interrupt behaviours that perpetuate depression and to develop a sense of power and self worth.

Physical activity: From adolescence onwards, women do less regular aerobic exercise than men, and therefore are less protected against depression. Assisting women who are slowed down by depression to increase their physical activity may be helpful. Women must choose the exercise that suits them, so that it is not yet another demand that cannot be fulfilled. Increased exercise on its own, however, is not a cure for depression.

Relationship therapy: Being in a relationship that is intimate, confiding and supportive seems to give protection against depression. However, married women have a higher rate of depression than married men. Working with a woman and her partner or family to improve their relationships may be useful. Individual therapy may reinforce the assumption that the depression is the woman's problem, rather than her way of coping, or her response to external stresses such as her husband's unemployment or her young children's demands for nurture. The family's expectations and demands for the woman to be a 'good wife and mother' will need to shift if she is not going to become depressed in future.

Family therapists examine the characteristics of what they refer to as 'depressed families'. Although it is much more common for female family members to manifest the depression, the depressed family itself uses certain social rules to govern beliefs and behaviour. Some of these rules include no direct expression of anger, a strong duty orientation, rewards for conformity, and punishment of spontaneity by shaming. Often 'helpful' behaviour on the part of family members exacerbates the woman's depression: trying to cheer her up may make her feel her depression is unjustified, while treating her like an invalid can perpetuate her 'sick role'.

Assisting and supporting women to leave destructive relationships may be appropriate in some circumstances. However, many women, especially those with young children, are constrained from leaving by financial and emotional ties. After separation or divorce, women, especially with children, are usually financially poorer than during marriage, and worse off than their former partners.

Group therapy: Group therapy has many advantages over individual therapy for depressed women. The support and understanding of a number of women militates against the 'patient–expert' relationship that exists to some extent in individual therapy, no matter how much the feminist therapist attempts to be open and equal with her client. Women learn from each other's experiences, and group experiences lead to the development of friendships that are essential for the prevention of future depression.

Self-help groups: Self-help groups are becoming more common and enable women to meet, share concerns and provide support and relief from the multiple roles they are expected to maintain. Women find that they are not alone in their experiences. They share, for example, the fact that bringing up children singlehanded is a very tiring and difficult task for anyone. Collective problem-solving and support encourage group members to take the risk of behaving in more personally satisfying ways.

Self-help groups break down the barriers experienced by many women in the therapeutic relationship, where the 'expert' health professional (usually male) treats his 'sick' patient (usually female). The vital principle in self help is that women are empowered by helping one another. Those who have worked through a depression can discuss how despairing they felt and how they eventually coped, guiding and supporting those women who are just starting to emerge from their depression.

Practical assistance: For many depressed women, therapy or self-help groups will not be available, or desired by the women themselves, especially when they feel particularly hopeless and helpless.

Helping a woman obtain some respite from her children, through occasional, overnight or daily child care, may be a first step. Informing a woman of her rights as a social security recipient, or tenant, or giving her support through legal advocacy so she can take out an intervention order against a violent husband, may be very important and life-changing steps.

Women from non-English speaking backgrounds may be informed about English classes. Older women may need assistance with meals and housework. Returning to education, or taking on part- or full-time employment can also often act to alleviate depression in women.

Structural change: We need to work together to make the health system more responsive to the particular needs of women by providing more opportunities for feminist therapy, better support structures, and more flexible treatment facilities (for example, where women may come with their children if they wish).

Women must be ensured adequate shelter and protection in a society which institutionalises violence against them, and disadvantages them educationally and economically. Major changes in the incidence of women's depression will occur only when women gain more social and economic equality. We need to work to change the social institutions which perpetuate women's distress.

References

Abramson, L., Seligman, M., Teasdale, J. 'Learned Helplessness in Humans: Critique and Re-formulation' *Journal of Psychology* 87, 1, 1975, 49–75

American Psychiatric Association *Diagnostic and Statistical Manual of Mental Disorders* 3rd edn, Washington DC; 1987

Berah, E. F. 'Sex Differences in Psychiatric Morbidity: An Analysis of Victorian Data' *Australian and New Zealand Journal of Psychiatry* 17, 1983, 266–73

Broverman, I., Broverman, D., Clarkson, F., Rosenkrantz, P. and Vogel, S. 'Sexrole Stereotypes and Clinical Judgements of Mental Health' *Journal of Consulting and Clinical Psychology* 34, 1, 1970, 1–7

Brown, G. and Harris, T. *Social Origins of Depression* London: Tavistock, 1978

Carob, A. *Working With Depressed Women* Aldershop: Gower, 1987

Edwards, A. *Regulation and Repression* Sydney: Allen & Unwin, 1988

Eichenbaum, L. and Orbach, S. *Understanding Women* Harmondsworth: Penguin, 1985

Grounds, David and Armstrong, J. *Ecstasy and Agony* (forthcoming)

McSwiggan, C. A., and Newgreen, D. B. *Nurses' Guide to Psychoactive Drugs* Sydney: Australian and New Zealand Book Company, 1982

Nairne, K. and Smith, G. *Dealing With Depression* London: The Women's Press, 1984

Rowe, C. J. *An Outline of Psychiatry* 8th edn, Iowa: W. Brown, 1984

Ryan, J. *Feminism and Therapy* London: Department of Applied Social Studies, The Polytechnic of North London, 1983

Seligman, M. E. P. *Helplessness* San Francisco: Freeman, 1975

Tinsley, E., Sullivan-Guest, S. and McGuire, J. 'Feminine Sex-role and Depression in Middle-Aged Women' *Sex Roles* 11, 1–2, 1984, 25–32.

Victorian Social Development Committee *Inquiry into Strategies to deal with the Issues of Community Violence: 2nd Report* Melbourne: 1988

Weissman, M. M. 'Sex Differences and the Epidemiology of Depression' in Howell, E. and Bayes, M. (eds) *Women and Mental Health* New York: Basic Books, 1981

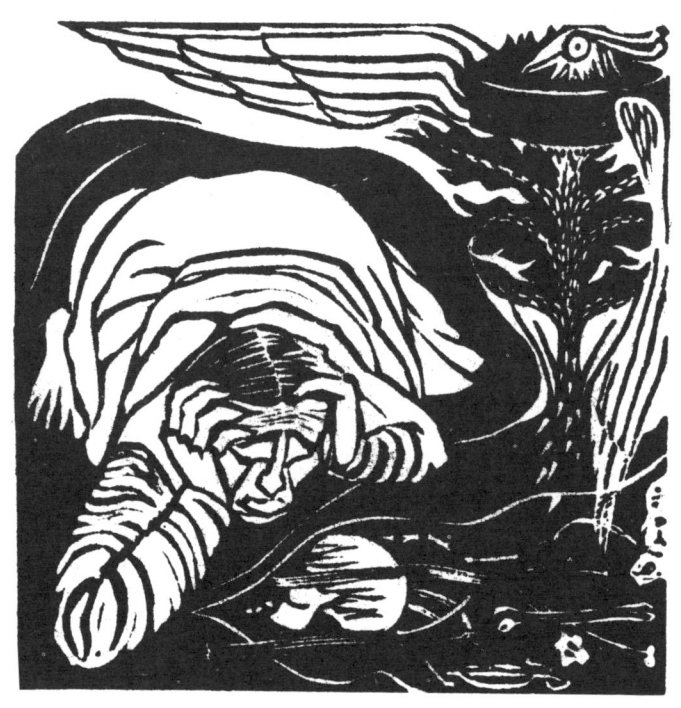

The Mill-stone, Judith Rodriguez

Rural blues

Gai Mayes

I have been married for seven years and have no children. I like to write and play music. My husband and I moved to the country for a more relaxed lifestyle. We never had a great deal of money but this did not deter us from our decision.

We moved to the local caravan park in which we were fortunate enough to have an understanding owner who waited, on occasion, a few extra days for the rent.

We were trying to make things work out, financially, emotionally and socially, but as hard as we tried things weren't going as we had planned or hoped. This I believe was the start of the corrosion of my self-esteem. Clothes were a complete luxury. It was totally out of the question to go and buy anything new at this stage. I felt my self-image was threatened.

After six months we found a house that suited us both very well. It felt like a real home. This I thought would be the start of another new beginning. But we had no car, no phone and no furniture. This was a downer to say the least. We did fix it up the best we could. Many times we went without food. After all the general household expenses, there was no money left.

Living out of town presented problems. I soon became used to long walks and all-day shopping expeditions. My moods at this stage swung from hopeful to hopeless. My husband's health made it impossible for him to work. I had been told jobs were hard to find, but I applied for work in various places anyway. I didn't get work.

Finally our resources were drained and we had to find some help with food and clothing. This was a very humiliating experience at the time. But the people who helped us were very nice and above all understood what we were going through. I'll always be grateful for the assistance they provided.

I was always worried about what would go wrong next. I was on edge a lot. Most of the time I was at home just waiting for the next pension cheque to come. It was practically impossible for me to communicate with anyone at that stage in my life.

I had been to the community centre a number of times for advice but I never seemed able to say how I was feeling or what I thought the trouble was. I guess it was a mixture of pride and still thinking 'everything will work out'.

When I was depressed, I felt I had to present a stable image on the outside, even though I was falling apart. There was no phone-line to call where someone would listen. I wish this had been available. I felt guilty because I wasn't managing. But it was a vicious circle. The more anxious I felt, the worse I managed.

I was feeling physically unwell nearly all of the time, and seeing the doctor on a regular basis. The reason I was feeling so sick, I told myself, was because of the house or even because it was a hot day. Any excuse came to mind. Eventually the doctor said it was my nerves. I couldn't accept this opinion because I felt physically ill. I felt desperate.

Then I began talking more with the women at the community centre. They were very supportive. This was my only contact with other people so their suggestions were important to me. I was given the opportunity of seeing a wonderful family therapist. I'll always remember her for her kindness and encouragement. These were the first steps towards recovery for me.

I was also able to attend women's groups and workshops as a community car was made available to me and other women who found themselves without transport. This was like being let out of prison. I became interested in things again and came out of my shell. But it took a great deal of time and effort to regain a feeling of well-being.

I met other country women who were depressed and that made me realise that many of us need emotional support at various times in our lives. We all suffered from isolation. For me, that meant I lost my sense of self-worth and self-expression. I was expected to blend into the background.

Women in the country are also starved for intellectual challenges. I would like to study, learn new skills and achieve things. There are a lot of women who are interested in the arts. But there aren't any outlets for exhibitions or musical concerts. This means both women themselves, and the community, miss out. Some women eat compulsively out of boredom and frustration.

Talking with other women has made me feel less lonely about living in the country. It no longer seems like an island. I felt trapped for so long, but now I'm trying to open up new and constructive activities for myself.

Part VI

The Quick Fix

Smoking
The pause that refreshes?

Lorraine Greaves interviewed by Linda Martin

Why do women smoke?

One of the functions of smoking for women is the actual suppression of emotions such as anger or fear. Women sometimes smoke instead of saying or doing something that might be disruptive to their family, or difficult to say, or not well received.

Smoking is also a way of controlling your social relationships. Women describe to me that they keep people away through smoking. They might say to their child, 'Don't bother me, I'm smoking.' On the other hand, it can also be a bond between people if both light up. It can be an equaliser.

What about women who smoke to keep their weight down?

Women think that if they quit smoking, they would gain weight. It's true to a certain extent, but after a few months it levels off. Smoking does suppress the appetite. I think there are a lot of young teenage girls in particular who are using smoking in that way.

What is the recent history of women smoking?

Cigarettes were first mass produced in the late 1800s, but they only became heavily consumed by women after 1920. So, it's a very short time in terms of our history.

In Australia about 28 per cent of women smoke. Is the rate similar in other countries?

Yes. In Canada it's about 30 per cent. In Britain it's higher. Certain countries stand out. Scotland, for example, has a higher rate of women smoking. But in most Western countries, approximately one-third of adult women smoke.

About 55 per cent of women smokers in Australia are in blue-collar jobs. Over 60 per cent have less than a Year 11 education. Can you talk about these issues?

Class, gender and race are the three factors that really describe the pattern of cigarette consumption across the world now. People with the least power are more likely to smoke. Added to that is the fact that young people, particularly young women, are increasingly likely to smoke. Of course, compared with males, females have much less power.

Has marketing played a role in encouraging women to smoke?

Yes, filter-tip, light, low-tar, low-nicotine, and long, thin cigarettes have all been created and promoted with women and girls in mind. In fact, low-nicotine cigarettes were designed to facilitate young girls' smoking, as they have lower tolerance for nicotine.

Are they actually less of a hazard?

No, and this is a real danger, because a lot of women believe that these cigarettes are less harmful and therefore a healthy alternative. But there's no such thing as a healthy cigarette.

Is there a danger level for smoking?

The more you smoke, the worse off you are. The conventional wisdom is that any consumption is dangerous. And only 2 per cent of smokers manage to keep it at a casual level anyway.

What about the dangers of second-hand smoke?

Passive smoke inhalation is a real problem. Long-term studies show that growing up in a smoking environment has an effect on children. Even if these children never smoke themselves, as adults they suffer from a greater incidence of chronic, obstructive lung diseases of all kinds.

You mentioned that young women are taking up smoking in increasing numbers. How do they get started?

When you ask women about their initiation into smoking, most recollect a social experience of some kind to do with their friends, or something that was a very vividly recalled rite of passage. I think that has a lot to do with why girls take that first cigarette.

The question is why some girls stop after that while others continue to smoke, because most children feel ill when they try their first cigarette. Part of it has to do with parental permission in the home. If there's actually a pro-smoking environment around the child, that makes it more acceptable. If you have to battle your parents to get permission to smoke, it's more of a deterrent.

Also, teenage girls begin to feel the pressures of growing up and being forced into stereotypical female roles. As I was saying earlier, smoking is sometimes an avenue for suppressing rage, fear or loss of control.

What images do advertisers exploit to attract women smokers?

The advertising images have remained fairly constant since 1920. Lightness, freshness and health have all been associated with cigarettes. Yet smoking actually has the opposite effect regarding any of these qualities. Smoking has also been conveyed as being heterosexually attractive. That women are tempted by these images just proves once again how powerful and seductive advertising can be. There was a brief theme in the 1920s and 1930s where smoking was promoted as a weight-control aid. An old ad was, 'Reach for a Lucky instead of a sweet'. The Confectioners' Association put a stop to that ad because they were afraid of losing business.

A familiar ad is the classic 'You've come a long way, baby' that associates smoking with women's liberation.

Cigarettes have been represented as a tool of emancipation. That ad for Virginia Slims started in the 1960s. It was most successful. They became a very large-selling brand of women's cigarettes. This ad suggests that women have achieved equality when in fact there are so many areas where women still have to struggle for their rights.

What other images are connected to smoking?

Women can appear tough depending on how they hold their cigarette, flick the ash or how they inhale. They can become very sophisticated depending on what kind of lighter they use or what brand they buy.

Some women roll their own. This might be seen as a statement that they are not buying into a prepared, commercial product. It's unfortunate, because these kinds of cigarettes are very dangerous. They're very strong and they're not filtered at all.

Are Third World women smoking?

In some countries, yes. It's determined, in part, by where the multi-national companies are. They're promoting smoking as a smart, Westernised thing to do. In some families that have a yearly income of just a few hundred dollars, from 30 to 50 per cent of that income is being used to buy cigarettes because of the dependence that's been created.

Also, land that is needed for food is being used to grow tobacco. It's similar to the Nestlé campaign in the 1970s for promoting baby food formula to women in Africa and developing countries. They try to push unhealthy and expensive products, that foster dependency.

The economic aspect of smoking is significant for women everywhere in the world. Most women make less money than men and can't really afford to spend any of their income on cigarettes. If you're spending money on smoking, you're not spending it on food, or transportation or education.

That's right. Some women talk in terms of $200 a month, which is a fair bit of money. But they don't have much choice over that spending once the dependence is established. Lower income women smoke to relieve stress, but smoking keeps you poor. It's a bit of a vicious circle.

Another key thing is time. Women spend about 200 minutes a day smoking. That's almost three and a half hours per day.

What are the health risks for women who smoke? In Australia close to 11 per cent of all cancer deaths of women are due to lung cancer.

Cardiovascular diseases such as heart attack and stroke are even more of a danger than lung cancer to women who smoke in Australia. They are the major causes of death. In the United States lung cancer is now the leading cancer cause of death in women.

Also, the links between smoking, cervical cancer and osteoporosis are ones which are just being recognised. The combination of birth control pills and smoking is another risk that is very frightening, particularly for women under 30.

Are women aware of these risks?

Yes, generally speaking. There are some issues like the cervical cancer and birth control pill risks that need more attention in terms of health promotion. What women are not aware of is that smoking is the leading cause of preventable death of women.

Women are in no way interested in killing themselves or depriving themselves of health. Many of the smokers that I speak to feel caught. They feel unable to extricate themselves from the dependency or from the situations that exacerbate that dependency.

You hear a lot about the effects that smoking has on the foetus. Is this a problem?

It's been focused on too much. It's been a major theme with respect to women through the anti-smoking campaigns, especially during the past ten years. 'Don't smoke when you're pregnant.' The second theme has been, 'Don't smoke because it will ruin your skin and give you facial wrinkles.' So women are viewed either as reproductive receptacles or nice-looking objects.

I'm not saying that smoking and pregnancy shouldn't get any more research attention. That should probably continue. But in terms of promotion programs, I don't think that we should be putting any money or effort into that theme for quite a few years to come.

In fact, I think it's been counter-productive. Women say things like, 'Oh, I quit when I became pregnant and I started again as soon as the baby was born' meaning that they would quit for an external reason, but not for themselves. One gets the impression that the woman's health isn't the important thing here—it's not worth quitting for. But the baby's health is, because the doctor says so.

It seems that many of the 'quit smoking' campaigns have put all the responsibility on the individual.

Oh, you're right. The campaigns have been badly worked, internationally. They have been misdirected. The idea that women are to be blamed for smoking is completely out of order.

The anti-smoking ethic adds to the panic of women who are dependent, and creates a self-defensiveness and guilt that I find really unfortunate. Women who are thinking of quitting benefit less from lectures on lung cancer than they would from being in a supportive environment that encourages them to develop a sense of power and self-esteem.

In my work, I never discuss cessation with women. What I discuss most of the time are their personal feelings about smoking and their interpretation of what it means to them. We do some speculation about what it might be like if smoking wasn't there. But that's it. Because to me, women as individuals or collectively will give up smoking when they feel more in control of their lives.

Smoking is actually a rational decision for certain women. And I encourage women to understand it that way sometimes. There are women to whom I would say, 'Don't try to quit right now. It has a certain level of importance at this point in your life, so weigh this up against what would happen if you tried to quit.'

There is a link between domestic violence and smoking. A lot of women that I speak to have been abused in relationships. They use smoking to hide their fear or to relieve stress. Often a cigarette becomes a barrier between them and a threatening man. Or smoking allows them to suck back their anger, which if displayed, could add to the volatility of a situation. In many instances where a man is an alcoholic or unemployed, the woman often bears the stress for the whole family. These are cases where smoking can be functional for women.

Do males and females have the same response to smoking?

In my work, I make certain that males and females are separated. Because so far there's been very little attention to women or girls per se, they've just been mixed in with men and boys. Quit smoking programs, and to some extent prevention work, has been very effective with males, but it hasn't been with females. This may be due to the fact that no one is really addressing the issue of sex discrimination and how it affects female smoking behaviour.

Are women trying to quit smoking?

Yes. About 95 per cent of the people who quit smoking, do so on their own and never really go to a group or any formal program. They have, however, absorbed certain materials or read certain literature. It is widely believed that women are less successful at quitting smoking than men. But that's really very difficult to prove. Some people suggest that if you added in men's pipe and cigar smoking, those rates would equalise. Also, the rates are often derived from looking at formal groups, and women are more likely to go to a formal group than men.

It's extremely difficult to quit smoking. Very heavy, long-term smokers actually suffer serious side-effects from withdrawal. It's been likened to heroin withdrawal with symptoms such as irritability, loss of ability to think clearly, anger, anxiety, lashing out emotionally and lots of crying. In addition, there are physiological symptoms like shortness of breath and pain in the lungs.

People try a variety of strategies for quitting ranging from nicotine chewing gum to self-help groups, to hypnosis and acupuncture. An interesting thing is that physician intervention alone can cause something like a 6 per cent quit rate, just by virtue of a physician raising the issue with the patient.

Do you think smoking should be banned or made illegal?

Well, lots of smokers think that, because it's a dependence and they welcome any external measures to limit their smoking. I don't think it's a practical alternative. It didn't work with alcohol many years ago, and it doesn't work with some illicit drugs. What is practical and reasonable is to ban the promotion and advertising of cigarettes.

What about designated non-smoking areas? Is this a possible compromise?

Yes, and I think the places where smoking is acceptable will become even more limited. There is increasing legislation that actually imposes fines on people who don't obey no-smoking regulations.

Is smoking perceived as a crucial health issue for women?

In terms of research, I don't think so. Often you'll read case studies about 200 male cardiac patients and then generalisations are made saying 'people' react in such and such a way. But 'people' really means 'men'.

One of the things that we have to do is to make women more visible. Yet women and smoking is even invisible within the women's health movement. Smoking is given low priority when, in fact, smoking kills far more women per year than other health problems.

Certain other substances like alcohol or heroin, if they are abused by women, often result in anti-social behaviour. As a society, we notice that and therefore we've given these problems some attention. Smoking does not create anti-social behaviour; in fact, it facilitates well-socialised behaviour in women. I'm suggesting that smoking is actually an instrument of social control of women, similar perhaps to minor tranquillisers.

My hope would be that smoking as an issue will be given priority in the women's health movement and that we recognise that this is another dimension of the victimisation of women. We need to take collective responsibility for raising awareness about smoking and lobbying for changes.

References

Greaves, Lorraine *Background Paper on Women & Tobacco* Ottawa: Health & Welfare Canada, 1987

Hill, David J. 'Australian Patterns of Tobacco Smoking in 1986' *Medical Journal of Australia* 149, 4 July 1988, 6–10

Jacobson, Bobbie *The Lady-killers: Why Women Smoke* London: Pluto Press, 1981

—— *Beating the Ladykillers: Women & Smoking* London: Pluto Press, 1986

Life on the wrong side of the scrim

My experience of benzodiazepines

Beatrice Faust

You asked about my experience of benzodiazepines. The first four encounters were trivial. The fifth was indescribably awful. I was prescribed Librium once for weeping and once for asthma. I was prescribed Valium once for asthma and once for anxiety. These drugs did me neither good nor harm and I stopped taking them after a decent interval. Then I took Ativan.

I could say that sinking into intoxication and struggling through detoxification was like playing my life always on the wrong side of a scrim. I could say that for five years I lived behind ambulance glass. In Boris Vian's play, *The Empire Builders*, there is a curious character, wrapped like a mummy, called the Schmerz—'pain'. His (or her) sole function is agonising. I could say that I became a schmerz—pained in body and mind because of a drug that assaults that nexus of mind and body, the brain.

Benzodiazepines have been the subject of major controversy ever since their introduction in the 1950s, stimulating Congressional hearings in the United States, and in Great Britain becoming the subject of the biggest round of litigation since Thalidomide.

It should be common knowledge that as little as one month on minor tranquillisers such as Serepax, Valium and Ativan can cause addiction, that addiction can sooner or later lead to complete physical and mental breakdown, and that withdrawal can be many times worse than withdrawal from nicotine or heroin—if only because it can take up to three years for the body's systems to regain their balance.

To become a benzo junkie is to become pain. That is the subtle effect. As for the crude ones . . . I had myself tested for diabetes and liver disease, syphilis and AIDS. There is no test for multiple sclerosis. By the time spontaneous bruising had become so obvious as to merit concern, I had discovered what was the matter with me— and it was not leukaemia. In between, I had a tooth restructured, had my eyes tested, my hip x-rayed, my abdomen palpitated and my womb curetted. I had an endoscopy and simple neurological workup. I tried to get a lithium test and a brain scan. I wondered if it could be Alzheimer's? A brain tumour? Bad genes? For over two years I was afflicted by a dreadful sense that something was wrong with me, and an obsessive determination to find out what it was. I went from a desultory pursuit of single symptoms as they arose to a frantic pursuit of 'it'.

I was told that I was malingering, hysterical, menopausal and . . . too clever for a woman. Having come through, I can assure you that benzo sickness is worse than benzo withdrawal and that withdrawal undergone with the support of kind, well-informed helpers is no harder than any other form of convalescence—every withdrawal symptom means that you are detoxifying and that is itself enough to let you experience the symptoms positively.

My story is very simple. In 1977, I was prescribed theophylline for asthma. It caused panic attacks but the benefit to my breathing, my sleeping, my arthritis and my spirits was so great that I clung to it, and tried to remedy the panic. I was prescribed Sematil, then Amitryptilline and Valium. No effect. I tried bio-feedback but that only worked when I didn't have a panic attack. I tried Ativan. It worked.

My story is very complicated. I was born with asthma and had probably developed bronchiectasis by the end of my first year. The scoliosis that I had developed by the age of nine or ten had become kaipho-scoliosis with osteoarthritis from the cervical to the lumbar vertebrae by the time I was 30. A psychiatrist once told me that, with my problems, I'd be crazy if I weren't depressed. However, I cannot explain my depression as simply a rational response to poor health. It is probably endogenous. There is alcoholism, suicide, depression, neuroticism and domestic violence in the three lines of my family that I know anything about.

I am not trying to speculate on my heredity but to show that the whole of my life has been passed in a state of ill-health and compliance with doctors. When the various symptoms of benzo poisoning emerged in relentless succession, I did not appreciate that they represented a new and vastly different problem from anything I had experienced. I had an existing framework to interpret them by. I explained the depressed breathing by the rotten state of my lungs, the joint and muscle pain by my arthritis, the lowered resistance to my general debility. The menorrhagia was ascribed to age and the emotional fog to the interaction of constitutional vulnerability with the stresses of being Beatrice Faust.

In 1982, when I began taking Ativan, I was 43. I had a rigid regimen that included about 40 minutes' yoga, 30 minutes' meditation, sundry pills and a compressed air pump to vaporise asthma solutions. I also had a disposition to keep regular hours and to eat whole foods as far as possible without being puritanical. I think this helped me to accommodate the benzo debility and to structure my life to withstand its undermining effects.

I had also, by then, endured five years of the anxiety that I called the Horrors. Kafka called it the Horror, Virginia Woolf called it the Fin. This began when I was prescribed a drug called theophylline for asthma. I would wake up—usually every second day but sometimes on consecutive days—overwhelmed by a sense of dread. It was as natural and inevitable as the rain on the roof. It was inside me. As I toughed it out, the tension would ease towards dinner time. On alternative days—sometimes for days together—I'd wake feeling buoyant, sanguine, my best self. Ativan erased all my pain and tiredness, sorrow and stress. Like a Bacchante, I laughed over my shoulder at my image in the mirror. I told my friends that I had discovered a wonder drug. That I would not be ashamed to stay on it for the rest of my life. That I had become whole.

How long did it last? I cannot remember. I do know that in 1985 I spent ten days in the world's second best hotel and that every other day I lived like an automaton—ventilated, exercised, showered, fed at regular intervals, and with the Horrors at my back. I thought it was because my marriage was breaking up.

The first symptom that told me I had acquired a new sickness was a dreadful stink. Initially, I thought it was the vaseline I'd been using to keep my leather dress supple. When I realised that it was in fact on my breath and in my sweat, I began a tedious round of doctors. Kind friends advised me to use perfume, drink lots of water, watch my diet. They placed me alone on one side of the dinner table, or invited me to take afternoon tea in the garden. Strangers recoiled and cruel people talked about me behind my back. The stink was actually a symptom of advanced intoxication. I had had earlier symptoms but had not recognised them.

The first was menorrhagia. My periods lasted as long as 23 days. The bleeding was so heavy that I felt as if I were passing a kilo of chicken livers, sensing large clots slipping through my cervix as quietly as ghosts. I bought Tampax and Modess in the largest sizes and the heaviest weights at Coles for efficiency and economy. The girls on the cash register used to cluck and coo as they handed me my parcel and say 'It's awful, isn't it?' Curettage and hormone replacement therapy did not help. I refused a hysterectomy and toughed it out until menopause supervened.

Next came nursing-mother randiness. My normal sexual style was masculine: I am visually aroused most of the time, although I have a weakness for vibrant voices and hair I can run my hands through. I prefer strong, intelligent, laughing men and athletic, performance-oriented sex. I expect every encounter to include at least one orgasm. That was transformed to a diffuse, never ending state of arousal, totally inward turned, without any urge to climax or, for that matter, any need to seek physical contact. I lapsed into fantastic dreams of romantic love—the most enduring being a passion for Tom Conti in his role as Colonel Lawrence.

Then my libido disappeared almost entirely. I both knew this was because of the pills and yet forgot the fact. At times I became a bit sad when I thought that the killjoys who said sex becomes boring if you have too much of it might be right.

A severe, unidentified pelvic pain became the third substantial warning that something was radically wrong. It was like an ectopic pregnancy. I thought that it might be an adhesion from my sterilisation. I did not ask how adhesions could appear after a ten-year interval. I thought it might be referred pain from my arthritic spine. Once more, investigations revealed nothing. Once more, I toughed it out.

Then came a series of little neurological symptoms—a tic in my left eyelid, clumsiness, dropping things and tripping over my feet. This went with an obsessive need to chew which I indulged by eating a packet of Vita-Weat at a sitting. (When the sickness entered its penultimate stage, this would turn into chewing cupfuls of uncooked rice.) No, I didn't have syphilis, and no, Ativan does not cause tardive dyskinesia. In any case, my symptoms were not the same kind of chewing as that melancholy disorder of the sedated aged.

I had an episode that looked like a slight stroke in which my right side was paralysed for a couple of hours. It was labelled Transient Ischaemic Anaemia. For over two years, whenever I bumped into people, or walls, or furniture, or fell over while getting out of a tram, I blamed the TIA. That's how I explained away biting my lips and the inside of my cheeks and becoming unexpectedly tongue-tied. I never asked how these symptoms could persist so long after their putative cause. Partly, I was set on being well, on functioning as best I could. Partly, benzos were making me slow-witted and passive.

I lost my concern for self-preservation and became enormously stoical, accepting risks and insults that would normally have stirred my adrenalin.

I had episodes of severely depressed breathing that were quite unlike either asthma or bronchiectasis. It was as if I kept forgetting to breathe. Since I could, by focusing my entire attention on that matter, force myself to breathe deeply and rhythmically, and since it did not escalate into an asthma attack, I tended to forget about it, except when I found that I could not control my breathing to lecture effectively.

My voice emerged flat and wooden and colourless.

This was actually the most serious of all my symptoms. People with bronchiectasis need to cough regularly or they drown in their own secretions. In hindsight, I realise that the prolonged and severe lung infections that caused me so much misery and were the despair of my physiotherapist were related to depressed breathing and the inability to cough. My poor paralysed lungs were breeding infection and I could not help myself by yoga or anything else. God knows how I survived.

I was beginning to look very ill. My hair became brittle and flyaway, my face became pudgy and my complexion dull. I stared into the mirror and looked for me in the image of the haggard stranger within my face. People started standing up for me in the tram. Gossips told each other that Bea Faust was getting seedy. Some of my friends thought I was dying.

I had the occasional hallucination—which I called optical illusions because they were so trivial and transient. I'd never tried hallucinogenic drugs and I had no frame of reference for these experiences. My vision became blurred and I fiddled interminably trying to orient my eyes and my glasses to read clear print. I quickly learned to make do with fuzzy. I felt enormous pressure inside my skull when I lay down to sleep. My limbs jerked in response to sharp pains, as if I'd been bitten by a giant stainless steel mosquito. Once I glimpsed the skin when this happened and the follicle had risen up like a huge isolated goose pimple—as if a nerve had fired randomly. I had a pain like barbed wire across my diaphragm and this did not relate to digestion or breathing. It was just a pain—nothing to take a pill for, but curiously unlike anything I had ever known. Nothing about benzo sickness or withdrawal is like anything I've ever known— although some other survivors say benzo withdrawal is near as a touch to the DTs.

'Oh sleep! It is a gentle thing. Beloved from pole to pole.' For years, I had used transcendental meditation to get to sleep. It had been a wonderful prophylactic. I told myself that the somnolence that increasingly overtook me was due to this facility developed by meditation. I fell asleep over the dinner table in Mietta's and told myself it was because I was bored by the *ne culturny* conversation of my husband's colleagues. Eventually, I was so worn down that I could prop myself anywhere and sleep for hours.

Sometimes, by contrast, I seemed to speed up, finding myself chattering maniacally. Or my handwriting would run out of control and crowd itself up into a corner of the page. I put too much chocolate in the mousse and had extraordinary difficulty following a knitting pattern.

I lost my sense of taste for many things and developed a curious catlike fastidiousness about food, unable to eat anything rich or greasy. This had nothing to do with nausea or gastric upset. It was a profound revolt against denatured food. I was more and more drawn to the simple subtleties of Japanese cuisine. I had a similar aversion to tea, coffee and alcohol.

These exquisite symptoms were accompanied by gross ones: my mouth sometimes filled spontaneously with viscous saliva—and I mean filled—I could spit half a cup or a wine glassful at a time. I also had a sensation as of moisture at the corners of my mouth. I dabbed obsessively when I was eating, but when I looked in a mirror for the dribbling there was nothing to be seen. My feet seemed to stick to the bathmat or the carpet even when they were quite dry.

I developed muscular stiffness and rigidity so severe that intercourse and even gynaecological examinations were difficult. Orgasm was terribly laborious and sometimes I suffered from cramps for as long as 30 hours afterward. It was as if any strong movement would lock my muscles in a painful after-image of activity. The muscles seemed to retain a chemical memory of what they had been doing. Occasionally, I'd be sitting in the tea-room talking about nothing in particular and I'd find my pelvis and thighs contracting orgastically.

Often the slightest effort was enough to give electric shocks to my joints. Guess how I explained those! I began to favour my limbs to avoid these various miseries. I disposed my body carefully when I sat down. I developed something that I called hard insomnia: it was as if every cell in my body was alert and defied sleep. Meditation did not relax me but I did it dutifully because I am a dutiful person and I was desperate. I judiciously used alcohol to get me to sleep—on good nights one ounce of spirits knocked me out. I never escalated that dose.

Nor, in all this time, did I increase my dose of Ativan. That would have been against my lifetime habit of following the instructions on the bottle. Since I related all my symptoms to other causes, I had no reason to use anti-anxiety medication for them. A friend tried to warn me that my pills were dangerous, and in my gullible arrogance, I assured him that lorazepam (Ativan) was not the same as diazepam (Valium). Neither of us knew that it is, in fact, much worse.

I knew that I needed my pills and that I'd suffer if I missed one but I thought that was because the absence of the pill simply revealed the presence of the problem it was meant to cure. I never considered that I might be addicted—not even after the time I missed a pill and woke up gaga. I read an article about pharmaceutical drug addiction but, since it was full of cliched human interest and had no salient information, I did not identify with any of the people interviewed. The significance of the discussion of Valium penetrated my stupor in a very peculiar way.

I somehow lurched through divorce and relocation. Finding myself alone on the first day of the rest of my life, I decided that I had no real excuse for being on happy pills. I halved my dose in March 1988. All of the neurological symptoms became worse. And the hallucinations. Life became anxiety. A simple photography review took three or four times as long as it should have. I knew that I had to do everything carefully or there'd be a dreadful snafu. I scanned my work for errors, I double checked. I organised my daily routine like computer programs so that everything led into everything else. I restructured my house to create a mnemonic web where I could shift things around so that they would be seen and not forgotten. I had always been the sort of person who made lists—shopping, things to do today, things to do next week. I depended on my lists. I used the kitchen timer to help me keep a real grasp on time.

I was beset by a prolonged, high-pitch ringing in the ears that lasted for almost a year. Flinders Street traffic at peak hour might drown it out and a couple of hours spent laughing with a friend could cure it for an equal period of time, but it seemed a permanent part of my life—indeed, it is not vying with the hum of the computer as I type. At times my eyes poured acid tears that dried in fine powder on my glasses. The ground undulated beneath my feet. I could not get my key into the lock without steadying one hand on the other. I became ambidextrous, making my left hand do more work because my right hand was doing less.

I suffered waves of weakness so great that a few coins placed in my hand by the market lady weighted it down like lead. I became paranoid, watching other people laughing and talking and imagining they were looking at me—just as people do in textbooks. I never knew when I picked my handbag up whether it would feel heavy or light. I became hypersensitive to noise and light. I saw myself living like an eccentric with most of the house in semi-darkness and silence, preferring to water the garden at night. I nearly ran out of *Ben Hur* but I was frightened of falling over the balcony of the Concert Hall in the dark. My skin would not tolerate the ribs on winter pantyhose or the weight of bedclothes. I dreaded shaking hands with people in case their fingernails brushed my skin. My own nails were pain enough. I drank compulsively and urinated to match.

All through this nightmare, words kept running through my head. 'I took Valium. It did nothing for me. I stopped it overnight. I am not an addictive personality . . . tried Valium . . . nothing for me . . . stopped overnight . . . Valium . . . overnight . . . not addictive personality.'

Somehow the penny dropped. It was not Valium but Ativan! I had been made a pharmaceutical junkie!

I rang the first emergency number I could find in the phone book—Alcohol and Drug Problems Direct Line. I had the best diagnostic interview I have ever enjoyed and within ten minutes I was in touch with TRANX (Tranquillizer Recovery and New Existence Inc.). It was nice to know I was not the only survivor, nice to discuss the dreadful business with others who had been there.

Soon after my first support group meeting, when I was having difficulty quartering a tablet, I gave up in rage and disgust. I threw the lot down the loo. I had been on 2.5 mg daily for five years and had come off in three and a half months. I'd kicked the habit practically before I knew that I had one.

Once I had a name for what ailed me, my symptoms became more manageable. I was not going mad. I was not going to die. I was going to detoxify.

My health returned even while the withdrawal symptoms were still unfolding. I became anorexic but energetic. I was restless and had brief episodes of agoraphobia, but my muscle tone improved and I stopped bumping into things. I tried to accelerate my recovery but found that there is no methadone for benzos. However, an article on radiation sickness yielded a thing that did give some relief: readily available amino acids and vitamins. I began taking tryptophan and nicotinamide and I recommend them heartily for anyone in the same situation.

Innocence gives me strength. Benzodiazepine intoxication is nothing to be ashamed of. It is not a matter of an addictive personality, but of pharmacological insult for which we are not to blame.

I consigned my benzos to the sewer in Spring 1988. I am writing this in Lent 1989. As I write, I have the sensation of something chewing my ear. It is a familiar sensation—almost friendly. The point about withdrawal symptoms is that they are signs of returning health.

Afterword—some facts about tranquillisers
Gwenda Higgins

In Australia it is estimated that one-third of the population has used minor tranquillisers at some time. In the year ending June 1986, the cost of drugs taken in Australia was 24 million dollars, with 5.87 million PBS prescriptions written. More than 70 per cent of tranquillisers prescribed are for women, and up to 18 per cent of women take one or more drugs on a continuing daily basis, compared with about 7 per cent of men.

The benzodiazepines (Valium, Librium, Serepax and the like) can cause dependency and withdrawal symptoms even when people take therapeutic doses (i.e. the amount prescribed). The major problem with dependence on minor tranquillisers is the process of withdrawal. For physiological reasons not fully understood, withdrawal is frequently a painful and protracted experience which may last for months or even years.

Doctors are often enthusiastic about recommending benzodiazepines and even encourage women to use the pills for long periods of time. Problems arise when women realise they are becoming dependent, or experience withdrawal symptoms or unpleasant side effects.

The influence of advertising by drug companies is also a major factor in the widespread use of minor tranquillisers. The profits from the sale of these drugs is enormous. Hoffmann–La Roche, the manufacturer of Valium and Librium, reported $389 million in profits in 1988. Valium was their second best selling product.

Doctors need to realise that prescribing a pill does not solve the social problems that women have to deal with. The answer lies in providing appropriate support systems for women so that they can feel valued and powerful.

References

Byrski, L. *Pills, Potions, People—Understanding the Drug Problem* Melbourne: Dove, 1986

Greenwald, John 'The Best Prescription' *Time* 4, 19, 8 May 1989, 62–3

Musgrave, A. 'The Serenity Pill' *The National Times* 6–12 April 1984, 18–19

Part VII

Violations

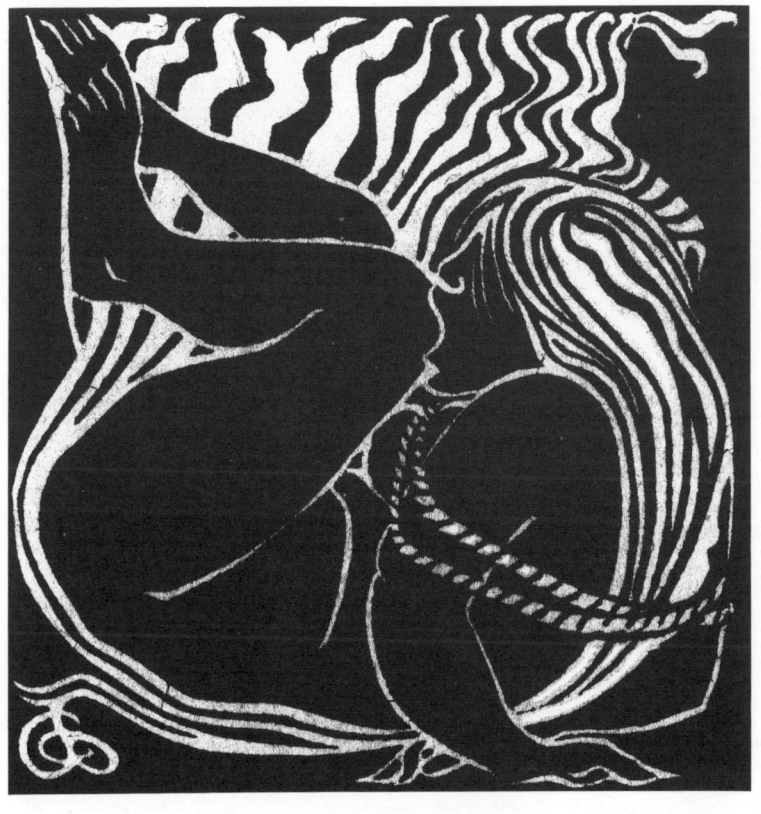

Water life, Judith Rodriguez, 1975

Sexual assault
More than a statistic

Diane Graham

(All names have been changed to protect the identity of the survivor)
Pieter became the love of my life, even though he had come to Australia for only six weeks. He also shattered my life; even today, I can't believe what happened.

I knew it would have to end when he admitted that he was married and his wife was expecting a child. But although I should have ended it all right then, I didn't. He went back to Denmark and we wrote each other hundreds of passionate letters. He kept saying that he was about to leave his wife. Eventually he did.

I went to Denmark to sort things out and ended up living with Pieter for six years. By then he had a little girl. I learned to love her although it wasn't easy. She was very insecure and there was incredible tension and guilt among the three of us. He spoilt her badly, and she was very demanding and often difficult, turning on temper tantrums when she couldn't get her way. I saw him hit her really hard several times; once he even kicked her. I was appalled. It was dreadful.

Yet to look at him you would never know he was violent. He was poetic, tall, thin, with long hair, gentle dreamy eyes and beautiful long fingers.

Anyway, in the end I realised I had to leave him because he wanted to have a child with me. I couldn't do it because of the way he treated his daughter. Things went from bad to worse. He made it very difficult for me to go. He would take time off work and just sit at home in the flat. I used to feel paralysed. He would just sit there. Eventually I was able to gather the strength to leave.

After I returned home we continued to write. It may sound stupid, but I tried to preserve the friendship out of past love.

Very early one Friday morning when I was in bed with my new boyfriend, the phone rang. It was Pieter informing me that he was coming to live with me. He was at the airport. I couldn't think properly.

I had no intention of going to the airport and I didn't. I was just about to leave for my teaching job when Pieter appeared at the door. He looked quite mad. He had everything he owned with him.

It was terrible. I really didn't know what to do. I had a sense of dreadful foreboding but tried to act as if I felt very secure. He was furious that I hadn't gone to the airport, and I couldn't make him understand that I had serious, important work to do and that I couldn't just take the day off, or I'd lose my job.

He wanted me to drink Galliano, there and then. He also wanted to go to bed with me. I absolutely didn't want to. He stripped off anyway. I was horrified. Semen began to drip from his penis and he accused me of making him spill his sperm and waste this precious commodity. I said, 'Look you're tired, you're overtaxed, sleep it off here.' Then I just bolted.

But I had to go back home after school. We began a huge series of debates. I tried to make him see that he couldn't expect to just walk back into my life like that, without it being my choice too.

He insulted me. 'You can't organise your own life. Someone has to organise it for you.' This was in spite of how much I'd done to separate from him and get my life underway again. He hit me over the head a couple of times, when I said something he didn't like. I really didn't know what to do. I just wanted him to get out. It was crazy and my mind was frozen, just frozen.

I'd asked my boyfriend Bill to keep right away, because I felt that I had to deal with it on my own. Bill was really very hostile about it, but he agreed to do what I asked.

Pieter became more rational and accepting during the weekend. I talked it through with him, and he seemed to be going along with everything. That's why I was lulled into a false sense of security.

On Monday morning, I remember saying, 'Well, I've got a lot to do today, what are your plans?' He said, 'I'll tell you what my plans are.' He reached over the side of the bed to a pile of things he had ready. Before I knew it, my hands and feet were tied and my mouth gagged. I tried to get up and fight. I freed one hand and put it under my back so that he couldn't get it again and I tore the gag off. He started hitting me over the head and calling me a bitch. I said, 'What, because I'm trying to get myself free?' And he said, 'Yes.' You know, in every way I felt more powerful than him, but he had the drop on me.

For hours he sat on me. He laughed and whistled. He smelled terrible and kept saying, 'You made me spill my sperm.' There was nothing I could do. Then he said, 'I've got a little surprise for you.'

I didn't know what it was, whether it was a gun or a knife or what, and I was so afraid.

I really didn't think I would ever get off that bed alive. I didn't dare scream. The only way out of it was to bottle it up. I knew from past experience that he got his cue from my reactions. I didn't want to trigger anything by losing my temper or screaming. It became really clear that I should do nothing. It's hard to say how long I lay there and how long he sat on me, whistling. Time seemed to stand still and I felt frozen. And I didn't cry . . . I just couldn't. I was totally paralysed but I knew I had to keep eye contact and I did. I looked him straight in the eye the whole time.

Eventually the phone rang. It rang, and rang, and rang. I kept saying, 'Look, it'll be my mother. She knows we're here and she's not happy about it. If I don't answer she'll send the police or my brother.'

The phone kept ringing and suddenly he said, 'All right, answer it.' I felt like I was floating up off the bed.

It was Bill. He sensed there was something wrong. I asked, 'Why are you coming round?' and he said, 'You're in trouble, aren't you?' I said, 'Oh, yes.' And he said, 'I'll be there in five minutes.'

I went into the lounge room, found some clothes that were lying around and got dressed. And I'd won, I'd won that round. I didn't leave the flat. I felt I couldn't. Everything I owned was in it and he was crazy enough to set fire to it, or smash things up. I felt that I could beat him just with willpower.

The next thing I knew he was standing in front of me flexing a whip. This was his 'little surprise'. I actually laughed, it seemed so absurd. That was exactly the reaction he was waiting for. He started whipping me. So, I did something really incredible. I pulled my hair back from my face and I said, 'Put one across there, and that will put you in jail. In this country that sort of behaviour is a criminal offence. Go, on. You just put one there and that's the end of you, mate.' He'd already whipped me across my arms and side. I had these huge weals around my wrist from the ropes too.

Bill arrived with some guys from work, and Pieter retreated to the bedroom. I rang the police. Soon the house was full of police and my brother arrived with his dog. My neighbours thought it was a drug bust and they ostracised me after that.

In the end, I dropped the charges, because I wanted Pieter to get out of the country. But he stayed around for six months, and during that time I lived with different friends. He kept leaving letters in my letterbox saying, 'Can't we just forget it ever happened and start back together again?' To this day I still get letters from him, which I never read. He even went to the Education Department and they very obligingly gave him the names of all of the schools where I worked. He followed me around and eventually I had to quit work.

My whole world was shattered. After the assault, everybody who knew about it saw me as a failure and a victim. In my brother's words I was 'a born loser'.

I went to Legal Aid for assistance. Finally someone suggested I contact WIRE [Women's Information and Referral Exchange]. They gave me a name and I had counselling for violent abuse. They also fixed up a solicitor, who eventually had Pieter deported. I also joined a group for survivors of sexual assault.

Although I am now in a mutually satisfying relationship, I still can't believe what happened.

The torture in rape and the rape in torture

Kate Gilmore

When women's concerns move into the public agenda, they have often been distorted or rendered 'gender neutral'. For example, violent assault against women in the home is frequently referred to as 'spouse abuse'.

Avoiding repetition of these patterns of distortion is the challenge confronting those who are concerned to ensure that women's experiences of sexual violence are not trivialised, and that the potency of the relationship between patriarchy, its masculinity and violence is acknowledged.

As women, we have little choice but to remain active and vigilant against sexual assault. This is not simply an honourable cause. This we must do if we are to be free from the threat, fear and actuality of sexual violence.

In reviewing the literature and statistics on rape, it may be said that sexual violence has been the experience of one in four women. Culture, ethnicity and class are not major factors in determining who will be a rapist. Most women are raped by someone they know, and it is not a 'crime of passion' but is usually premeditated.

Sexual assault is conventionally seen in terms of the individual rapist's or victim's behaviour—for example, 'she was asking for it' or 'he was provoked'. Thus the social or historical context is not taken into consideration. The conventional view supposes sexual violence to be the product of promiscuous or frigid women, sexually extravagant men or primitive heterosexual instincts.

Radical feminist theory offers a different explanation. In her book *Against Our Will*, Susan Brownmiller wrote: 'Rape . . . is nothing more or less than a conscious process of intimidation by which all men keep all women in a state of fear.'

The most generous of Brownmiller's critics have suggested hers is a position which is guilty of 'oversimplification' and a 'historical generalisation'. Less kind are those who have chosen to typify her contribution as that of a 'raving, bra burning, ball-breaking, man hating, reactionary'.

There can be no question that of the two explanations for sexual assault, the feminist interpretation, while being the most concerned with gender, has remained in the margins of contemporary thinking on violence.

To be of pragmatic value, explanations of sexual assault must use images and concepts which speak to the majority of people (women and men) while not blunting or muting the truth. Explanations must bring meaning to those who themselves have been sexually assaulted and must point forward towards change which will achieve the goal of prevention/elimination of sexual assault.

The relevance of torture

Perhaps most immediately relevant to this task is an emerging body of literature and research concerning the experience of torture survivors. This work describes social and political functions which torture serves in countries which are under the control of totalitarian regimes. The research and theories on torture may also be relevant for a social analysis of rape.

Not insignificantly, many victims of torture, and in particular women torture victims, are sexually assaulted as part of that experience. In fact, it might be claimed that the socio-political function served by sexual assault in contemporary Western, 'democratic', patriarchic capitalism is similar to that which torture serves in totalitarian regimes.

The question is how to assess this claim for both accuracy and practical value. A case for accuracy can be built in the five areas which follow.

Definitions: The World Medical Association, in its 1975 Tokyo declaration described torture as: 'the deliberate, systematic or wanton infliction of physical or mental suffering by one or more persons acting alone or on the orders of any authority to force another person to yield information, to make confession or for any other reason'.

The World Health Organization (WHO) (1985) defines organised violence as:

> the interhuman infliction of significant, avoidable pain and
> suffering by an organized group according to a declared or
> implied strategy and/or system of ideas and attitudes. It
> comprises any violent action which is unacceptable by general
> human standards [sic], and relates to the victim's feelings.
> Organized violence includes, inter alia, torture, cruel, inhuman or
> degrading treatment or punishment . . . or any other form of

violent deprivation of liberty also falls under the heading of organized violence.

The notion of intent contained within the Tokyo Declaration, its description of the torture agent and his motives, does not exclude from its umbrella sexual assault as it occurs in 'democratic' society.

The WHO definition focuses on 'organised' violence and emphasises the notion of 'avoidable' pain inflicted by a group organised according to a declared or implied 'system of ideas and attitudes'. If we accept that sexism is such a system of ideas and attitudes, and that sexual assault is a form of 'cruel, inhuman or degrading treatment', then rape is as much 'organised violence' as torture is. The definition of torture also refers to 'any other form of violent deprivation of liberty'. Isn't this relevant to the systematic deprivation of women's rightful freedom to move safely through the streets at night?

In 1988, writing under the heading 'Torture as the Perversion of a Healing Relationship', Schlapobersky described torture as 'an intimate and intense relationship between an individual and one or several others'. He compares the role of the torturer to the role of healer. Both have intimate contact with another's mind and body, but while the healer comforts, the torturer destroys.

Rape too is an intimate and intense relationship. The rapist and lover can also be compared. And it is the rapist who perverts the trust, confidence, intimacy and function of a consensual sexual relationship.

Sexual assault as a technique of torture: 'Torture almost always includes humiliation in the form of sexual abuse.' (Roth, 1987)

'The last mentioned (i.e. sexual torture) is of course, a form of physical torture but the psychological element will always overshadow the physical. Sexual forms of torture include verbal humiliations, being forced to undress in front of the guards, being forced to sexually satisfy a prison guard . . . as well as actual rape and/or violence to the sexual organs.' (Lunde, 1982)

The research on torture techniques, which documents the frequent application of 'sexual torture', thus reveals the extent of the torturers' confidence in the effectiveness of sexual violence. The spectrum of these sexual torture techniques demonstrates the torturers' understanding that effective sexual torture includes a continuum of techniques from verbal harassment to 'actual' rape. Feminists have long used a notion of continuum to describe the links between a 'wolf whistle' and a 'rape'.

However, it is a quote from authors Buus and Agger which best exposes the power of sexual violence: 'An important aim of psychological torture is to break down the identity of opponents, making them politically impotent so that they are no longer a threat to those in power . . . This is done by aiming the torture at the opponent's most vulnerable personal points: their sexuality and gender identity.'

This acknowledgement takes us to a point of convergence with the 'radical' Brownmiller assertion. For here are conventional medical model researchers emphasising that 'political impotence' meaning an absence of 'threat to those in power', is achieved 'by aiming the torture' at 'sexuality and gender identity'.

This may represent a new level of insight into the role and function of sexual violence in contemporary, patriarchal democracy. Perhaps Buus and Agger help us to see that the continuum of sexual violence has, as a consequence, the political control of its victims. Even if this is not the formal, organised or overt intent, perhaps it is the consequence.

If Buus and Agger are correct, the medium of sexual violence is actually a most powerful means by which the securing of submission and compliance can be attempted, and thus the political status quo protected and maintained. This analysis may mean that in Western democracies the sexual abuse of women and children (i.e. non-men) is designed to ensure that the existing male power base is not threatened.

Consequences for victims/survivors of rape/torture: 'Most victim/survivors (of torture) experience mental symptoms as being more disturbing than physical injury'. (Lunde, 1982)

Although the extremes of physical pain and subsequent long-term damage are not as common for the victim of sexual assault as for the victim of some forms of physical torture, the persistence of 'psychological' consequences is similar. These include nightmares, sleep disturbance, persistent fatigue, headaches, inability to concentrate, appetite loss, diffuse muscular pain and memory loss.

In social terms, consequences can result in family and friendship disintegration, social isolation and alienation, or a feeling of social inadequacy or incompetence. In material terms there could be a significant loss of economic status due to inability to work, loss of 'attractiveness' to employers, transfer from place of usual dwelling, from country of origin or of temporary residence. There is also the possibility of depression, anxiety, self-hatred, guilt, despair, diminished self-confidence, deep self-doubt and sexual disorientation.

As is the case for victim/survivors of sexual violence, torture victim/survivors struggle with intense feelings of guilt and self-disgust. While both the act of torture and the act of rape are dependent on rendering the victim 'utterly powerless and helpless', the victim will often hold herself/himself responsible.

Each will re-examine time and time again, her/his life up to the point of the assault/torture, seeking to identify alternative choices which, if taken, would have guaranteed a different outcome. Each will re-live, through nightmare, flashbacks and memory, the detail of the assault/torture, punishing herself/himself for not 'resisting' more, for not 'co-operating' less, for 'having given in'.

The notion of 'silence' plays a significant role in the experience of both the torture and sexual assault survivor: 'Many victims have told us that they felt so humiliated under torture they thought they would never be able to tell what really happened.' (Genefke, 1984)

'For centuries women have kept silent about rape and other violence out of fear and isolation.' (Sydney Rape Crisis Centre, 1984)

Crucial to ensuring this silence is instilling the conviction that no one else will believe you:

'Indeed we think that there is a myth surrounding torture, created by the torturers who try during the torture to induce so much suffering, humiliation and guilt into the victim that they would never be able to explain their suffering to other human beings.' (Genefke, 1984)

Rapists, too, so that their crime will not be revealed, use shame and threats such as 'they'll know you asked for it; they'll know you're dirty; they'll know you like it; don't tell anyone or I'll come back for you or I'll kill you.'

The titles of key texts on sexual assault emphasise the central role played by 'silence'—for example, *Women's Silence, Men's Violence; Conspiracy of Silence; The Best Kept Secret; I Never Told Anyone.*

Genefke describes the power of 'silence breaking': 'When the victims contrary to the wish of the torturers, start trying to explain what they have been through, the myth is broken . . .' This is exactly the message of the women's movement when it calls for the 'breaking of silence'.

Similarity in support services: The torture literature and the feminist literature on sexual assault promote similar principles on which support services should be established. For example, with regard to medical 'treatment', the torture literature emphasises:

1 All procedures which may cause uncontrollable pain and memories are systematically avoided
2 Precise information about all aspects (of the service) must be given and (the survivor) must fully understand and accept all procedures
3 It is of the utmost importance that the therapist (including physician) is never identified with the aggressors (torturers). (Somnier and Genefke, 1986)

In the development of feminist-oriented services to victims/survivors of sexual assault, these emphases translate, literally and symbolically, into a priority concerning:

1 promotion of the rights of the victim/survivor to choice, option and control
2 provision of comprehensive, accurate and accessible information concerning procedures and rights
3 consent of the victim/survivor to all procedures

So as to avoid identification with the aggressor, feminists have argued that the gender of all support workers (particularly those involved in the provision of medical services) must be other than that of the offender (i.e. not male).

With regard to providing support to rape victims, the worker must ensure 'problems are interpreted in a social political framework without denying the individual situation of the particular woman' (Lowenstein, 1983).

When working with torture victims, Buus and Agger state that the ideology of the support worker affects 'treatment, outcomes and processes of the psychological integration'. They suggest that the key elements of psycho-therapy for the torture victim include:

1 testimony and externalisation
2 reframing and validation
3 deprivatisation

In regard to *testimony* and *externalisation*, Genefke says: 'We stress very much that the victim, as soon as is possible, should talk about the detail of the torture and the suffering to which she/he has been exposed.'

The feminist movement has also stressed 'speaking out' or 'breaking the silence' or 'naming the experience'.

With regard to *reframing and validation*, Bloch says the victim of torture must receive external validation so as to reveal that 'it is the perpetrator (not the victim) who has violated his own humanity and dignity'.

Genefke emphasises that support provided must affirm that 'the victim's reactions . . . are consonant with the healthy person's response to something which is incredible, atrocious and perverse: torture'. Feminists have called this 'normalisation'.

In regard to both torture and sexual assault, emphasis is placed on the issue of guilt. The therapeutic response must show the victim/survivor that 'whatever happened during a torture session, the guilt is uniformly on the side of the torturers and the repressive system using such methods. The victim can never incur guilt in a torture situation'. (Genefke)

Somnier, writing in 1987 in the *British Journal of Psychiatry*, says, 'it is emphasized that a victim cannot have responsibility for what he [sic] did in a situation of utmost physical and psychological pain'. This is what the feminist movement means when it says, 'No excuses, never, ever!', emphasising the necessity of locating full responsibility back with the offender.

With regard to *deprivatisation*, emphasis is placed on the exploration of links between the individual's experience and the socio-political context in which the torture or assault took place. The argument in favour of such a process is put by Buus and Agger. They criticise traditional treatment for 'directing victim anger against the torturers (alone), rather than against the system which created the torture and to which the (tortured) is opposed. Using this approach torture and perpetrators become isolated from the political struggle which was the underlying cause of the torture. This might contribute to the (survivor's) feeling of the meaninglessness of the pain experienced.'

If, as Buus and Agger assert, 'The intention of psychological and sexual torture is to convert, symbolically, political strife into internal personal strife', then the therapeutic process must ensure that the connection between personal experience and political circumstance is re-established. This is again an essence of feminism made famous through the tenet, 'the personal is political'.

Role and function of torture and sexual assault: 'The victims of torture are always individuals but never individuals alone. The suffering of the individual is the torturer's access to the community.' (Schlapobersky)

'Torture is used to terrorize opponents and the whole population.' (Pagaduan-Lopez)

'Rape is a form of mass terrorism.' (Griffin)

'Men use rape as a means of direct control over women.' (Clarke)

'It is not nature that has constructed this effective system for the subordination of women. The system is constructed by men, in men's interests, for the benefit of all men.' (London Rape Crisis Centre)

The intention of both sexual assault and torture is to render powerless and politically ineffective its potential challengers, through making an example of individual victims.

Practical implications: Sexual assault continues unabated. Although it is only recently that its incidence has begun to be revealed, its prevention is far from assured. At the very least the concept 'torture' provides a metaphor for sexual assault which accurately communicates the reality of the sexual assault victim's experience to a society which still believes rape is enjoyable.

The comparison also furthers the struggle for an analysis of sexual assault which is relevant across cultures and encourages a consideration of gender in the research of torture.

It points to the hypocrisy, if not the outright racism and sexism of Western governments. They condemn the 'third' or 'under-developed' or 'eastern bloc' world for human rights violations. Yet sexual assault in their own countries is tacitly sanctioned or dealt with ambivalently by the legal and social systems.

Perhaps the imagery of torture comes closest to communicating to men the full impact of what is the primarily female experience of being raped.

Conclusion

'When people who have endured a nightmare begin to talk about survival, it behoves us all to take account of what they say.' (Schlapobersky)

The public domain of decision-making and cultural gatekeeping—the politicians, senior bureaucrats, the judiciary, the faces behind big business—by any measure is overwhelmingly male and overwhelm-ingly influential. The paradigm of 'torture' may provide another string to our bow in the fight against trivialisation of violence to women. It may help us listen to the 'speaking out' of both the tortured and the raped. It must help us join together in the struggle for universal human rights, a struggle which must address gender and rape; which must not presume torture is something which only happens in other countries; which recognises the torture in rape and the rape in torture.

References

Amnesty International *Torture in the Eighties* London: 1984

Bloch, S. 'Interrogation and Torture' in R. Bluglass (ed.) *British Textbook of Forensic Psychiatry* London: 1988

Brownmiller, S. *Against Our Will: Men, Women and Rape* London: Secker and Warburg, 1975

Burgess, A. and Holstrom, L. 'The Rape Victim in the Emergency Ward' *American Journal of Nursing* 1973, 1740-5

Buus, S. and Agger, I. 'The Testimony Method: the use of therapy as a psychotherapeutic tool in the treatment of traumatised refugees in Denmark' *Refugee Participation Network 3*, November 1988

Cathcart, L. M. et al. 'Medical examinations of torture victims apply-ing for refugee status' *Canadian Medical Journal* 121, 12 July 1979

Cienfuegos, A. J. and Morelli, C. 'The testimony of political repression as a therapeutic instrument' *American Journal of Orthopsychiatry*, 53, 1983, 43–51

Clarke, A. *'Doctors, Ethics and Torture'* conference held in Copenhagen, August 1986

—— *Women's Silence, Men's Violence* London: Pandora, 1987

Genefke, I. and Aalund, O. 'Rehabilitation of Torture Victims' *The Danish Medical Journal*, January 1983

Genefke, I. 'Rehabilitation of Torture Victims' paper given at *The Violation of Human rights: the quest for understanding* conference, California, 22–23 September 1984

Griffin, S. *Rape: The Politics of Consciousness* San Francisco: Harper and Row, 1986

Health, Political Repression and Human Rights conference held in Costa Rica, agenda for 26 November 1989

Kordan, D. K. et al. *Psychological Effects of Political Repression* Buenos Aires: Planeta, 1986

London Rape Crisis Centre *Sexual Violence: The Reality for Women* London: The Women's Press, 1984

Lowenstein, S. F. 'A Feminist Perspective' in A. Rosenblatt and D. Waldrogel (eds) *Handbook of Clinical Social Work* San Francisco: Jossey-Bass, 1983, 518–48

Lunde, I. 'Mental Sequelae to Torture' *Danish Medical Journal*, August 1982

Pagaduan-Lopez, J. C. (ed.) *Torture Survivors: What can we do for them?* Manila: Philippine Action Concerning Torture, Medical Action Group Inc. 1987

Rasmussen, O. V. and Marcussan, H. 'The Somatic Sequelae to Torture' *Danish Medical Journal* March, 1982

Roth, E. et al. 'Torture and its Treatment' *American Journal of Public Heath*, 77, 11, November 1987

Schlapobersky, J. 'Torture as the Perversion of a Healing Relationship' paper given at American Association for the Advancement of Science conference, Boston, February 1988

Schwendinger, J. and A. *Rape and Inequality* Beverley Hills: Sage Library of Social Research, 1983

Shapcott, D. *The Face of the Rapist: Why Men Rape—the Myths Exposed* Auckland: Penguin, 1988

Somnier, F. E. and Genefke, I. K. 'Psychology for Victims of Torture' *British Journal of Psychiatry*, 149, 1986 323–9

Sydney Rape Crisis Centre *Surviving Rape* Sydney: Fontana, 1983

Wilson, E. *What is to be done about Violence Against Women?* Harmondsworth: Penguin, 1983

It's been a long road
A women's crisis centre in Fiji

Shamima Ali

Early in 1983 in Suva, Fiji, a non-Fijian woman working with the government was raped by two men who broke into her house where she was alone at night. A police spokesman at the time of the incident told the press that there had been quite a few cases of rape that year and there was little the police could do about it. He added that police believed the men in this case had watched the woman undress before they entered the house. He said that in some rape cases women had 'tempted men by undressing in a room where they could be seen from the street' and in others by 'going out alone at night'. 'We appeal to women to take more care,' he said.

This incident acted as a catalyst to a group of women who had already shared their feelings of concern at the frequency of sexual attacks on women in and around the city, and the total lack of any support services for the victims. They met and resolved to work towards providing such a service.

Today in Suva, the Women's Crisis Centre occupies four rooms in the front part of a house in a prominent section of the city. This is a far cry from 1983, when the centre occupied two small rooms in the back street of the city. The centre is open five days a week from nine to five, and on public holidays and Saturday mornings.

It has been a long road between that first informal gathering of women and the existence of a functioning centre today. The members of the Women's Crisis Centre say the road ahead will be longer. A great deal has been achieved, but we feel we have only just begun to make our mark.

Initially the aim of the group was to provide a service for the victims of rape. However, the more the women looked into the issues involved in rape in Fiji, the more aware they became of the magnitude of violence against women generally, particularly domestic violence. They broadened their charter and services are now available to all women and children who have suffered violence at the hands of men.

The centre offers services which are typical of any rape crisis centre, including self-defence classes. It also offers crisis intervention measures appropriate to other types of violence, including finding a safe place to go and legal assistance. (The public legal advisor is a woman and also a member of a sister organisation, the Fiji Women's Rights Movement.) We are at the moment in the process of developing an extensive community education program and conducting research into the circumstances and magnitude of violence against women in Fiji.

The membership of the group has changed too, since those early days. It is no longer a group comprised mainly of women from overseas. There are now 21 of us, mainly local women. The centre is no longer staffed entirely by volunteers. Due to an increase in client numbers, it became absolutely necessary to employ full-time staff at the centre. There is now a co-ordinator, a clerical assistant, a research/education officer, a full-time and a part-time counsellor, and we are in the process of employing two more part-time counsellors. Each member undergoes a counsellor-training program. The centre operates as a collective. We have maintained a democratic process of policy- and decision-making. We hold regular workshops to review our work and to discuss issues that concern the centre.

The women at the centre bring to the group not only a rich variety of cultures and races, but different backgrounds, philosophies and motivations. Reasons for volunteering vary and include religious commitment, commitment to feminism, personal or close experience of violence, simple abhorrence of violence against women, strong aversion to injustice, or a combination of all these factors. The centre functions with remarkably little disharmony. It seems that any philosophical differences have become unimportant in the face of a shared concern.

There is little doubt of the magnitude of the problem of violence against women in Fiji. No very recent figures are at hand, but since the coups there seems to be a significant rise in the number of cases of violence against women, particularly gang rapes. No figures are currently available on the incidence of prosecutions in cases of domestic violence. Statistics on domestic violence are being collected by our research officer. We believe that the incidence of unreported attacks is quite likely to be even higher than in developed countries because of the norms of the Fijian and Indian cultures. A lot of women commit suicide because of unbearable domestic violence which they cannot escape.

The Women's Crisis Centre is the first and only organisation providing non-judgemental assistance to the victims. There are no refuges or women's homes. It is very difficult for women to leave their marriages. The only government support for women on their own with children is a destitute allowance of $40 per month. It is very rare to get even this, and funding sometimes runs out.

The two military coups in Fiji have worsened the situation of women in the country. Vanessa Griffen has written:

> The political, economic and social effects of the coups are a national problem; women are the victims in some areas more than others. The obvious areas are those based on their sex: sexual abuse and rape are increased risks for women in a state such as Fiji's at present; women's traditional role in the family also means they bear the burden of feeding families when jobs are lost and money is scarce; as low income and non-unionised labour, women are the hardest hit by wage and job cuts.

The Women's Crisis Centre has had to set up an emergency fund to aid starving families since all welfare agencies are filled to capacity. The emergency fund has also enabled children to attend school and women to receive medical treatment.

At its setting up, the centre had hoped to have some influence on the judicial procedures which, in Fiji, are behind those in most developed countries. For example, non-molestation orders do not exist, and if there is a dispute between husband and wife, the magistrate's duty is to promote reconciliation. The victim's past sexual experience is still admissible evidence in court, rape within marriage is not recognised as a crime, and sentencing is far from befitting the crime. For example, in 1982 'A 22-year-old man in Nadroga admitted raping a four-year-old child left alone in a house while her aunt and a friend had gone out to a dance. The man had broken into the house and raped the sleeping girl. He was sentenced to three and a half years in gaol.' In 1988 two youths who raped an eighteen-year-old girl were given two and a half years' suspended sentence in the High Court by Chief Justice, Sir Timoci Tuivaga. The two pleaded guilty. Passing sentence, Tuivaga said it was unusual for the court to give a suspended sentence for such a serious charge. But he said the circumstances showed the girl lived a 'loose form of existence'.

Because of the strain on our womanpower at the centre, we talked about a sister organisation which would look into the judicial system. In April 1986, some crisis centre members with some members of the YWCA formed the Fiji Women's Rights Movement, which lobbies for law reforms and which acts as a watchdog for any sort of sexist and discriminatory actions against women in the media and elsewhere.

Since the centre's opening in August 1984 until early 1989, we have assisted over a thousand cases, mostly of domestic violence. Although this number may not appear large, we strongly believe that this is a significant response in a society with no previous orientation to this type of service.

We also believe that a much greater use of the centre's services will result, as more funding and more personnel will enable us to publicise the centre more widely. The centre has as yet no established ongoing source of funding. We have existed on donations from foreign embassies, business houses, concerned individuals in the community and small government grants. A substantive grant was requested from the United Nations Fund for Population Activities (UNFPA) but the government aid co-ordinating body (whose members are all male) turned the proposal down twice, despite letters of support from other welfare organisations in the community, and despite our personal submissions. The reason for the refusal was never given to us but we learnt later that they did not approve of the word 'Crisis' in our name—it gave Fiji a bad image!

At the moment, the UNFPA proposal is with the Ministry of Women and we are awaiting endorsement of it. Our financial situation has improved tremendously through substantive grants in 1987 from the Regional YWCA, the Canadian High Commission in Wellington, and from the Australian International Development Aid Bureau (AIDAB).

We are now once more seeking funds for 1990 and after. Funding agencies are reluctant to fund salaries, but they do not realise that without staff, the crisis centre cannot remain open. We are also looking for funds for a refuge for women. This is a gigantic task but we are willing to tackle it because the need is so great. Acceptance into the community has been slow—a lot of people see us as radical, anti-family feminists. We at the centre say that in a country where bureaucratic processes are particularly cumbersome and life moves at a pace called 'Fiji time', where education standards are low, sexism is hardly subtle, and consciousness of personal rights and expectations of justice are lower than those in developed countries.

Perhaps two of the most important things we have learnt from our experience are patience and persistence. Despite all the difficulties and setbacks, we are still here. More and more women are using our services and we have no doubts about the value and survival of the Women's Crisis Centre.

References

Action Centre for Women in Need *Rape in Fiji: a Preliminary Report*
    Suva: 1983, 5
Fiji Times, 23 February 1988, 2
Griffen, Vanessa Women and the Coups in Fiji, unpublished paper

Part VIII

It's a Test

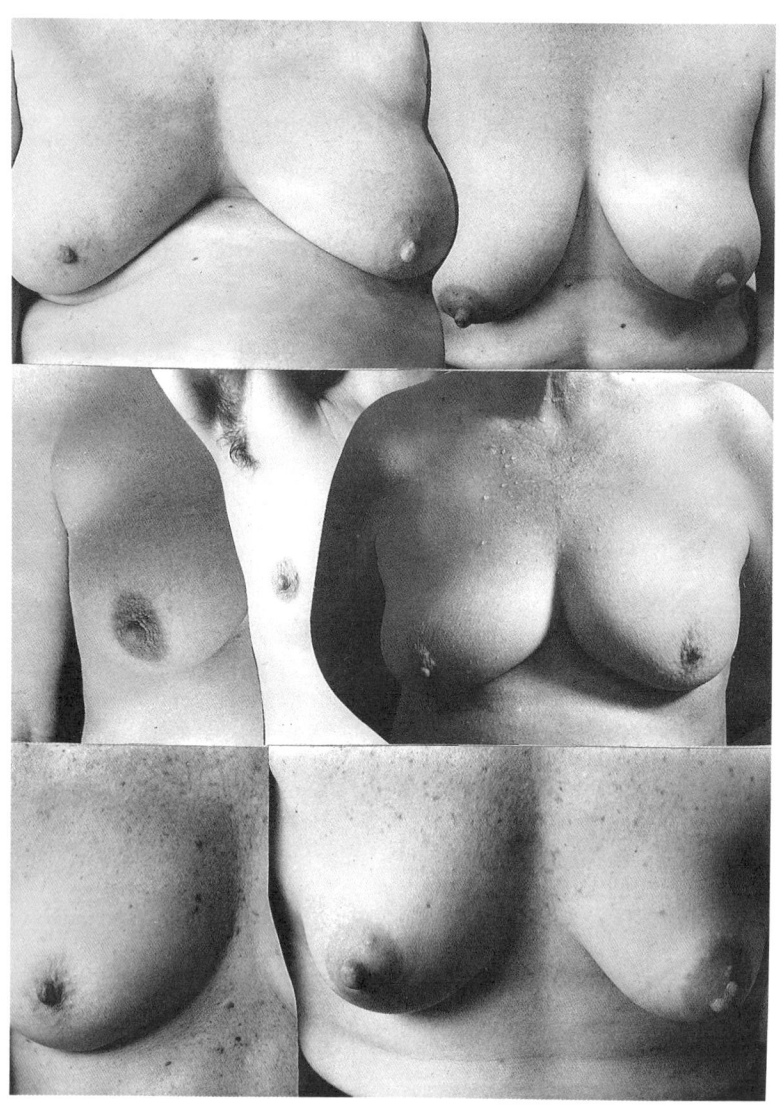

Breast collage, Joyce Agee, 1989

Taking control over technology

Screening for breast cancer

Sandy Gifford

It was a Sunday afternoon in late October when I first interviewed Mary, a 45-year-old woman who had recently been diagnosed with breast cancer. At the time of the interview, Mary was undergoing chemotherapy and was recovering from surgery. She explained to me that she had discovered a lump in her breast while showering:

> I was just taking a shower and instantly I felt total, total panic. My heart raced. I thought 'Oh my God!' You know, 'I'm too young!' I didn't want to think about it . . . and all day I just carried it around, all tight and panicky, and I thought about . . . I thought about the articles I had read that said the worst thing you can do is not confront it . . . [you should] go and see someone. It's that fear that leads to so many deaths . . . The strange thing was, I was finally feeling good! I felt better than I had in years! I felt terrific! You know, I had come through all these bad periods from February to July and then I felt really good. The world looked wonderful and then all of a sudden, I got the news . . .

Perhaps one of the most distressing aspects of breast-cancer is its invisibility, the lack of symptoms in its early stage. Often, by the time a woman does become aware of symptoms, it has progressed to a stage where her life is in danger and extensive treatment is recommended.

It is precisely this problem that has led to the development of technologies that can be used to screen healthy women in order to detect early breast cancer. The rationale behind screening is that if the cancer is detected in its very earliest stage, before a woman has any symptoms, then treatment is less dramatic and a woman's chances of survival are increased. Thus, for many women, taking part in breast cancer screening programs may result in longer and better lives.

However, a major factor in ensuring that screening technologies benefit women is to make sure that they are used appropriately. Like all technology, breast screening, if misused, can cause more harm than good. Thus it is important that we as women learn how to take control over these technologies so that they work for us and not against us.

The aim of this article is to assist women to become better acquainted with breast screening so that, if they decide to take part in screening programs, they will be able to gain maximum benefit from the results. I have divided this article into two parts. The first section briefly describes the problem of breast cancer. The second explains the kinds of breast-cancer screening technologies available, the risks and benefits of mammography and how individual women can increase their chances of having 'good' results if they choose to be screened for breast cancer.

Why is breast cancer a problem?

Most of us are well aware that breast cancer is the leading cause of death and illness due to cancer among women. The number of new cases of breast cancer per head of population has risen somewhat over the last twenty years, while mortality (death rates) has remained about the same. The reasons for the increase in the number of women who get breast cancer are not well understood. Some researchers believe that it is partly because more cancers are being detected in their early stages. If this is the case, then we would expect to see the number of cases level off over time. However, other researchers believe that the increase is real.

A major problem with breast cancer is that the causes are unclear. Epidemiologists who have studied the occurrence of breast cancer in large populations of women have discovered a number of risk factors that appear to be associated with the disease. Before discussing these risk factors, I feel it is important to first examine what is meant by the concept of risk, as it is commonly misunderstood by both women (as clients) and medical practitioners alike. A risk factor is something that appears to be associated with an *increased probability* of the occurrence of a disease.

The important thing to keep in mind when discussing risk factors is that they are determined by studying large populations rather than individual women and they do not establish cause. It is always difficult to translate risk factors derived from large populations to a specific individual. So, when an individual woman is told that she has risk factors for breast cancer, she must remember firstly, that her risk is not the same as for a larger population; it may be more or it may be less. And secondly, she must remember that risk factors do not establish cause.

The major risk factor for breast cancer is age: a woman's chances of getting the disease increase over the age of 45 years. This means that every woman is, to a greater or lesser extent, at risk of developing breast cancer as she becomes older. A second major risk factor is her family history. However, the link here seems to be strongest with women who have a first-degree relative such as a mother or aunt who developed breast cancer in both breasts before menopause. Studies have also shown that women who had their first pregnancy over the age of 30 years show an increased risk. However, groups of women who have never become pregnant seem to be at a lower risk than those who became pregnant for the first time after they were 30. Breast cancer appears to be more common among women who eat high-fat diets and also among women in the upper socio-economic groups.

Until recently, benign 'breast disease' was thought to be a risk factor for breast cancer. However, pathologists are discovering that there are many different types of benign conditions and most simply represent a range of normal changes within the breast. Many doctors now argue that it is incorrect to diagnose many benign changes as a disease because 'lumpy breasts' may be normal for many women. The real risk for many women with lumpy breasts is that they or their doctor or other health-care practitioners may fail to detect a lump that does need further investigation. However, because a few types of benign conditions may eventually become cancerous, it is important for women who have a biopsy to have a clear understanding of the diagnosis and prognosis. Finally, it is important for women to realise that factors which may cause many benign breast lumps may not be the same factors as those associated with cancer. For example, many doctors believe that caffeine can cause breast lumpiness and advise women to cut down on the amount of caffeine in their diet. But caffeine has not been shown to be associated with breast cancer, so women should not assume that by cutting out coffee or tea, their risk of developing cancer will be lessened.

So, while researchers have been able to discover a number of risk factors for breast cancer, no one has been able to pinpoint the cause of the disease. In fact, it may well turn out that there is no single cause. Thus a woman's age is the best predictor and since all women get older, it is very difficult to define a single group of women who are at high risk.

The above problems explain why much of the emphasis on controlling breast cancer has been through secondary prevention and mass screening. Let us examine each of these strategies separately. Primary prevention involves strategies to prevent a disease from occurring in the first place. However, primary prevention can only be carried out when we know the cause of a condition and when we have the ability to remove the factors in the environment that expose individuals to the causal agent. Because we do not as yet know the cause of breast cancer, the best we can do is to detect it early so that further illness and death can be avoided. Secondary prevention is directed at reducing illness and preventing death through early detection and prompt and effective treatment.

Screening is a strategy aimed at secondary prevention and is offered to 'healthy' people who do not as yet feel ill. It is not diagnostic in that a screening test does not indicate that an individual has a disease. Rather, it can simply separate those individuals who probably do not have a disease from those who may have it and so need further investigation. There are different kinds of screening strategies and the best strategy is to screen only people who are at high risk of developing a disease. This is often referred to as 'the high risk approach'.

However, as we have seen with breast cancer, it is not possible to define a single group of women who are at high risk. All women are at some increased risk as they get older. Because of this, the approach most used with regard to breast cancer involves mass screening where all women over a certain age are invited to participate. Thus, when we speak of mass screening for breast cancer, it is important to keep in mind the following points:

1 Screening is aimed at healthy women.
2 Screening is not diagnostic; it only separates those women who probably do not have the disease from those who may, and who need further follow-up.
3 Further follow-up may be indicated when the tests themselves are wrong (e.g. the technology has not functioned properly) or when a symptom is detected that needs further investigation.
4 Further follow-up often involves repeating the screening test or undergoing further tests which can diagnose the disease.
5 Screening cannot prevent breast cancer from occurring; it can only prevent further illness and death.

What kinds of breast cancer screeening technologies are available?

There are three types of techniques that have been used most frequently to screen women for breast cancer. They are a breast self-examination (BSE), a clinical examination of the breast by a doctor or other medical practitioner, and mammography. Each of these techniques can play an important role in helping to detect breast cancer, but only when they are used appropriately.

I shall begin by briefly discussing mammography, primarily because it has received a lot of publicity over the last two years and many medical practitioners and women are looking to mammography as the answer to breast cancer. Mammography is an x-ray of the breast and, until recently, it has been used primarily as a diagnostic technology. That is, a woman was referred by her doctor to a radiologist for a mammogram only if she was at high risk or already had symptoms for breast cancer. However, mammography cannot be considered to be truly diagnostic because the only way that a doctor can be sure that a woman has breast cancer is to do a biopsy, that is, remove some of the suspected tissue and look at it under a microscope. Thus mammography has traditionally been used as one of a series of steps in the diagnostic chain.

One of the advantages of using mammography for screening healthy women is that it can detect tumours when they are still too small to be felt by a medical practitioner or by the woman herself. Several recent studies carried out in Sweden and in the United States have shown that, when used to screen women over the age of 50 years, mammography can help to reduce deaths due to breast cancer by up to one-third. Some more recent evidence suggests that screening with mammography is also of benefit to women between the ages of 40 to 50 years but this is still an area of considerable controversy.

There are two main reasons why mammography is not as effective in younger women. Firstly, their breasts tend to be denser and it is more difficult for the mammogram to 'see through' the tissue and pick up tiny tumours. Secondly, breast cancer tends to develop more rapidly in younger women, and thus there is a shorter time period before cancer symptoms can be detected.

Finally, mass screening has been shown to be less effective in women over the age of 65 years. The reason for this is that in order for mass screening to be 'cost effective' the majority of eligible women must be willing to participate. However, studies have shown that it is difficult to encourage women over the age of 65 years to participate in screening programs. Additionally, breast cancer is less aggressive in older women and a woman's chances of dying from another disease, such as heart disease or stroke, are much higher.

There are two major benefits to women who choose to participate in a well-conducted mammography screening program. Firstly, for those women who are found to have breast cancer, some will benefit by having their life extended through early detection and treatment. Unfortunately, not all women will benefit in this manner. However, all women who have been found to have cancer should benefit by being able to choose a less radical treatment and by having a greater choice of treatment options.

Unfortunately, there are also risks to women participating in mammography screening programs. Mammography is not 100 per cent accurate, and this means that results can turn out to be falsely positive or falsely negative.

A false positive result occurs when a mammogram is interpreted as abnormal but upon further investigation it turns out that the woman does not have cancer. False positives can occur for many reasons. In new programs, the radiologists who read and interpret the mammograms may not be experienced and thus they are more likely to err on the side of caution. Older machines or machines not designed specifically for breast screening may also give false results.

There are many different kinds of tissue changes that occur in the breast, most of which are normal and are not cancerous. However, it is sometimes difficult to distinguish a benign or harmless change from a malignant change until some of the tissue has been analysed in the laboratory.

A major problem with a false positive result is that in addition to the anxiety it causes women, it can lead to unnecessary biopsies. While needle biopsies are sometimes possible, other biopsies require minor surgery and can result in pain, discomfort and in scarring of the breast. New programs typically have higher false positive rates when compared with older, more well-established ones. However, the false positive rate should drop over time as the operators become more experienced.

Mammography screening programs can also produce false negative results. This occurs when the mammogram is interpreted as being normal when, in fact, a woman does have cancer. The reasons for a false negative result are similar to the reasons for a false positive result and include inexperienced operators and machines that are not designed to pick up small tumours or changes in the breast. In addition, some women's breast tissue may be too dense and thus tissue changes are not easily detected.

As the above discussion suggests, it is important for women to understand that mammography screening is not foolproof. The technology is not necessarily the whole answer to the problem of breast cancer. However, a high quality, well run mammography screening program may help to increase both the quality and length of the lives of women who develop cancer.

There are many components that make up a good mammography screening program. Here I shall discuss only a few of the key components. Firstly, it is essential that screening services use a dedicated mammography machine that is designed according to current standards and delivers the lowest possible dose of radiation. Older machines used to deliver relatively high doses (2–3cGy), but newer machines should deliver between 0.05 and 0.15cGy. When properly used, the risk of getting breast cancer from the new low-dose machines is much less than the risk of getting 'naturally-occurring' breast cancer.

Secondly, it is important for the service to employ a radiologist who has a special interest in breast cancer. This is because the interpretation of a film that may be abnormal is a developed skill. One radiologist whom I interviewed explained:

> This [radiology] is not a perfect science. There are errors involved. Some cancers just don't show up and sometimes they look as though they're benign and some benign things are malignant . . . It requires our experience and expertise in looking at these images and saying 'There's an area I'm concerned about or that's not one I'm concerned about.' A great deal of it is subjective. It's much more an art than a science I think. The interpretation of mammograms are based on experience . . . So you really need a combination of technically good images and an interested interpreter who has had some experience.

Thirdly, ongoing evaluation and assessment of the interpretation of films must take place. Radiologists should check each other's work, and films of women that were interpreted as negative but who later developed cancer should be compared to ensure that an early cancer was not missed.

Fourthly, a multidisciplinary team consisting of a clinician, a radiologist, a pathologist, an oncologist and a nurse should carry out the assessment of screen-detected abnormalities. This is an essential prerequisite of a screening service in order to ensure that women receive appropriate follow-up and diagnostic services and that they have a choice about treatment if it is needed.

Fifthly, it is essential that counselling and information be readily available to women. Health-care providers specially trained in breast health should be available to explain the screening procedure, answer questions and discuss possible outcomes with women at the time of screening. The same individuals should be available to answer questions, provide information about the results of the test and to inform and counsel women if they need to return for a repeat screen.

If the woman needs further diagnostic follow-up, counselling and advocacy should be provided to ensure that the woman and her family receive appropriate information and advice concerning follow-up and treatment options. It follows that in multicultural communities, these services should be developed taking into account language and other cultural factors.

Finally, it is important that screening programs are not discontinued once women have initially taken part. Although most will have a negative result, this does not mean that they are free of cancer or that they will not develop cancer in the future. Programs have an ethical responsibility to ensure that women who wish to continue to be screened at appropriate intervals have access to such services.

Many women and medical practitioners have expressed doubts about the effectiveness of breast self-examination (BSE) and thus may look towards mammography as the technological answer. However, there are several important reasons why breast self-examination should continue to play an important role in the early detection of breast cancer. As we have seen, mammography is not very effective at detecting early cancers in most women under the age of about 40 to 45 years. Even if it were effective, the routine exposure of younger women to x-rays may have harmful health effects. One of the benefits of BSE is that women themselves can become familiar with what their breasts 'normally' feel like, so that if anything out of the ordinary occurs, they can seek further medical follow-up. However, for many reasons, some women may not wish to examine their own breasts on a regular basis and instead may wish this to be done by other health-care providers, such as doctors or nurses.

A physical examination by a health-care provider is an important screening technique, especially for younger women. However, the ability to carry out a thorough examination is an acquired skill and health professionals receive little training in breast care. As a result, many may not have the skills to conduct thorough examinations. One clinician experienced in carrying out breast exams explained to me: 'Well, there is a feel, just an instinct when you know, if you've felt a lot of breast lumps. There are things that I feel confident about that are movable, rubbery, they're symmetric . . . I put a lot of credence in my fingers . . . '

It is important for women to make sure their health-care provider is experienced in carrying out a breast examination, and this is not an easy task. One way is for women to learn how to do a BSE and then to ensure that the clinical examination is at least as thorough. Another way is for women to sit down and discuss the clinical examination with the health-care provider. Health-care providers who specialise in women's health may also be more skilled in carrying out examinations. Finally, it is essential that more emphasis be placed on the training of primary care providers so that they have the opportunity to build up their skills and expertise in the art of breast examination.

Taking control over breast screening technology
As we have seen, there is no foolproof method of detecting breast cancer in its early stages. There are, however, several technologies, including mammography, breast self-examination and clinical examination, that can benefit us. As discussed, these technologies can either

help or harm us, depending on how they are used. The important point for women to remember is that we must to some extent take control over the available technology by asking questions and making ourselves as informed as possible about both the risks and benefits. This is not always an easy task. Two women I interviewed explained:

> I just had a physical last week and I did tell my doctor about this breast lump. Why is it that I come across doctors that are not providing a little more thorough breast examinations? . . . It's frustrating. He said, 'Oh, I don't feel anything.' But he didn't show interest . . . I feel a little like I'm sort of on my own with this thing.

> I think they (the doctors) ought to make what they're talking about clearer because it took me a long time to understand . . . They tend to talk around you, like you're . . . you know . . . an idiot! I find that many times doctors talk to women like they're stupid . . . They think we're too emotional.

While it may be difficult for women to challenge health-care providers by asking questions and making choices based on information received, it is important that we have the courage to do this, for if we do not, the technologies that are designed to help us may end up causing us more harm than good.

References

The Breast Cancer Digest Bethesda, Maryland: National Cancer Institute, 1984

Fentiman, I. S. 'Pensive Women, Painful Vigils: Consequences of Delay in Assessment of Mammographic Abnormalities' *The Lancet* 7 May 1988, 1041–42

Forrest, P. *Breast Cancer Screening: Report to the Health Ministers of England, Wales, Scotland and Northern Ireland* London: Her Majesty's Stationery Office, 1986

Gifford, S. M. *The Meaning of Lumps: A Case Study in the Ambiguities of Risk and Benign Breast Disease* PhD dissertation, San Francisco: University of California, 1986

Hall, F. M. 'Screening Mammography—Potential Problems on the Horizon' *New England Journal of Medicine* 314, 1986, 53–5

Hutter, R. V. P. 'Goodbye to Fibrocystic Disease' *New England Journal of Medicine* 312 (3), 1985, 179–81

Last, J. (ed.) *A Dictionary of Epidemiology* New York: Oxford University Press, 1983

Love, S. M., Gelman, R. S. and Silen, W. 'Fibrocystic "Disease" of the Breast: A Non-Disease' *New England Journal of Medicine* 307, 1982, 1010–14

Mitchell, H. 'Organized Mammographic Screening Programmes: A Benign or Malignant Neglect?' *The Medical Journal of Australia* 146, 1987, 87–90

Mueller, C. B. 'Surgery for Breast Cancer: Less May Be As Good As More' *New England Journal of Medicine* 312 (11), 1985, 712–13

Skrabanek, P. 'False Premises and False Promises of Breast Cancer Screening' *The Lancet* 10 August, 1985, 316–19

Shapiro, S. et al. 'Ten to Fourteen-Year Effect of Breast Cancer Screening on Mortality' *Journal of the National Cancer Institute* 69, 1982, 349–55

Tabar, L. et al. 'Reduction in Mortality from Breast Cancer After Mass Screening with Mammography. Randomised Trial from the Breast Cancer Screening Working Group of the Swedish National Board of Health and Welfare' *The Lancet* 1, 1985, 829–32

Something happened on the way to the orifice
The vaginal examination

Discussion between Rose Sorger and Jan Southgate

Rose: Jan, you have recently completed a report for the Health Department on how to teach medical students to do vaginal examinations. Your study involved public hospitals, and as a part of your research you spoke to health workers. What were some of the experiences they told you about?

Jan: One was about a fourteen-year-old girl who came to a counsellor in a very distressed state. She had been to the hospital because she thought she might be pregnant. She was examined by a doctor in the presence of six students! No fourteen-year-old can give adequate informed consent for students to be present. Obviously this girl was anxious when she went to be examined. Certainly she had enough to deal with, without having an audience as well.

I've also spoken to many nurses, and they really know what goes on in hospitals. Some have been very upset about things they've seen and heard. One student nurse witnessed a medical student carrying out at least eight pelvic examinations on women who were under anaesthetic for other surgical reasons. They certainly hadn't been admitted for any gynaecological difficulties. The incident was reported to one of the teaching staff.

Another shocking incident happened to a young woman of nineteen who came to the hospital for a gynaecological problem. She undressed and her legs were placed in stirrups. She had to wait for quite a while until the doctor arrived and when she was examined, five medical students were present, plus a nurse.

Once the doctor had examined her, he proceeded to discuss her case with the students while the woman was still lying on the table and in stirrups. He said to the students that this medical complaint was common in promiscuous women. He then went on to ask her whether her partner was a married man, and how old he was. Following that discussion, the doctor actually slapped her on the thigh and left the room! That really reflects pure sexism in its worst form.

Rose: Yes, those of us who have worked in public or private hospitals can recall many examples of indignities that women have suffered when having vaginal examinations. I have seen women complaining bitterly and getting absolutely nowhere. And doesn't the example you have given demonstrate how doctors and other health professionals can be extremely judgemental regarding women's sexuality? In my experience as a nurse, I've also seen women in outpatient departments of hospitals being told to undress, don a backless gown and climb onto an examination table often without the curtains being closed. People passing by in the corridor can see in. This is very demeaning.

Jan: A lot of women have had that kind of experience and they just won't go again to be examined because they do not want to be put in that position. All dignity is lost. People enter cubicles without asking or looking in to see if it's occupied. Women may be left uncovered on examining tables. There is just no basic respect.

Rose: I've noticed medical students and doctors approach women with a great deal of apprehension. One can sense they have a certain amount of dislike or fear of women's bodies, in fact the women can often see this reflected in their faces. The women themselves are also feeling very anxious about the vaginal examination. They worry they are sweaty, or smelling unpleasant, or that an infection is noticeable. I think there's a real separation between the woman and the medical student or examining doctor. There's fear on both sides, but different fears.

Jan: This is something that's just not addressed in medical teaching. Nowhere in the course do they sit each student down and say, 'How do you feel about touching a woman's vagina? Are you apprehensive? Let's talk about it.' They are virtually put to the test in practical circumstances within the hospital. But of course, once the examination is underway, there's no opportunity to deal with feelings of aversion. Even afterwards the student can't say to the consultant, 'I had difficulty with that,' because it would be seen as a weakness.

Rose: Is there an attempt to discuss unconscious fears and ambivalence towards women's bodies or resentment of female sexuality?

Jan: As far as I know, medical school courses don't acknowledge these attitudes. We also have to remember that a lot of medical students are young people who have come straight from school to university. They've possibly had very limited life experience, so one response is to try to desensitise themselves so that the vaginal examination becomes a very cold, clinical procedure.

Rose: Also, I'd say that a number of doctors who are teaching students are unsatisfactory role models. Students may come in and be greeted with, 'What have we got here, another gynaecological voyeur?' I mean, the woman and the students who hear this don't know how to respond. Medical students can learn some very dismal habits from some of the more arrogant, insensitive doctors.

I remember a woman coping with the struggle of recent migration from Scotland who had come in to be examined. The gynaecologist spent most of the time while he was examining her bewailing the cost of Scotch whisky and the cost of private school fees as well. He thought he was being quite sociable.

Jan: Some doctors tend to think that by talking about the football and anything other than what's happening to the woman, she will feel more comfortable. Obviously this is not the case. Actually the doctor probably feels more comfortable if he doesn't have to explain the procedures, while most women would prefer to hear what the doctor is about to do next and why.

Rose: This inability to communicate is even worse when the examination takes forever. Some women endure one examination after another with no chance to object to the procedure. In obstetrics, students are being trained to determine the position of the baby in the uterus. They do a manual examination through the dilating cervix by trying to feel the soft spots and suture lines where the skull bones join in the baby's head. This is difficult to pick up and so they often have to keep trying repeatedly. The doctor is standing at their side demanding, 'Can't you feel it? Can't you feel it?' I have seen women suffer in these circumstances but they are totally ignored.

Jan: Many women giving birth aren't consulted about having student involvement until they are actually in quite heavy labour. At that stage they are so involved with what is happening that they are not in a position to give true informed consent. It is usually after the birth that they often feel they have been violated.

Rose: And this is just one example. Sometimes the vaginal examination is so rough that women cry out in pain. Women can be reprimanded for complaining or asking that students not be present. The stock response is that students must be trained.

Jan: Most women really have no knowledge of their rights within public hospitals. And public hospitals are not all that keen for women to know their rights. There is an impression that because public hospitals give free service and are teaching institutes, women have to accept students being present or examining them. But this is not so. Women have the right to refuse.

Even highly educated women who may be assertive and know their rights find that they are more vulnerable in either private or public hospitals. When you are lying naked and perhaps not feeling well then it is hard not to feel intimidated by doctors or other authority figures.

Rose: So women must be backed up by policies and protocols where the onus, the responsibility, is on the hospital or the physician not to infringe on a person's rights. Do you think patient advocates are effective or sufficient?

Jan: I think one advocate in any hospital will not always be available when a patient needs their assistance. They'll never be able to give one-to-one service. A patient advocate should have to be like an equal opportunity officer who establishes policies and practices that are in patients' interests.

Furthermore, the advocate would be a hospital employee and answerable to hospital administrators. This makes it more difficult to side with a patient against the hospital or against doctors. Nurses are often expected or willing to take on the role of patient advocate. But again, they don't have the power to initiate changes.

Rose: I have often been struck by the fact that, during a vaginal exam, doctors rarely ask women what experiences they have of their own bodies, or tell women what is going on. And for women with limited language skills or from various cultural backgrounds, a lack of interpreters or understanding by the health professional offers even less opportunity for communication.

Jan: That's right. And perhaps they don't want to give women that knowledge. But doctors can't learn much either without getting information from the woman. Yet they don't see health care as a partnership and they assume that women don't know much. Of course, for women of non-English speaking background all these problems are magnified. Interpreters are needed and are not easily available.

Rose: Women often want more information about infections or changes in their cycle and try to talk to doctors about self-help measures, nutrition or stress in relation to menstruation or recurring vaginal infections. But usually doctors won't spend time on these matters.

Jan: Yes, these questions are often regarded as tedious. And I think this is still the case in general practice and in hospital clinics. One of the big complaints from women is of poor communication. Doctors would gain a wealth of information if they actually asked a woman about her body. But there's a whole new breed of doctors now who are interested in community health and preventive care. Maybe that's a sign of things to come. We can only hope.

Part IX

Begat, Begotten and Bewildered

Hanging out the cradle
Early midwifery

Helen Myles

The history of childbirth is largely a woman's tale, but until recently it has usually been related in terms of the male history of the medical specialties, obstetrics and gynaecology. An 1872 history of English midwives, written by a man, set the tone for the historical format. It stated that 'the dark ages of midwifery' might have continued for many years if 'men of high social and medical position' had considered the study and practice of midwifery 'beneath their dignity'.

Examination of birth practices before the European settlement of Australia is useful, because the British and American experience prior to this time provides knowledge of the background and influences brought to Australia by early white settlers.

Throughout much of history and in many cultures, women have controlled their own reproductive activities, and women have been recorded as midwives from the beginning of history. In almost all early depictions of birth scenes, from crude cave drawings of the ice age to the elaborate sculpture and delicate details of the Renaissance, the attendants are women. It was women who were the early healers, using remedies devised from commonsense, experience and superstition.

The 'sage-femme' or 'wisewoman' of the village is reputed to have had skills in anatomy, physiology, astrology, psychotherapy and pharmacology. She is also known to have used painkillers, digestive aids and anti-inflammatory agents. Belladonna, digitalis and, in the midwifery field, ergot (to prevent bleeding after delivery of the placenta) were commonly used remedies.

The word 'midwife' has the literal meaning of 'woman who is with the mother at birth' and an earlier English meaning, 'woman who pulls the baby out' is still used in some cultures today. Other common terms for midwife are 'with-woman', 'good woman', 'cunning woman' and 'wisewoman'.

The early midwife combined a series of skills, superstition and comfort techniques when attending births. She is noted to have coaxed the baby out with singing and chanting or stroking, and to have administered herbal remedies to the mother throughout labour. Her main expertise lay in severing the cord and delivering the placenta if necessary. From time to time the midwife may have examined the cervix to gauge the progress of labour, but mostly she comforted the mother and directed the liberal fortification of the labouring woman with herbs, hard liquor or mulled wine.

Podalic version (turning the baby in the womb) had been practised by midwives from the first to the eleventh century. However, during the Middle Ages, midwives feared the use of version, for if the baby died or was born malformed, the midwife was at risk of being branded a witch and executed. So this form of interference, albeit a skill for midwives, ceased to be used by women attendants.

Midwives were usually older women—preferably those who had also experienced a number of births themselves. They were therefore able to offer advice from their personal as well as their professional experience. They would also have witnessed many births, for it was traditional for a woman to call her friends and relations into the lying-in room during labour to watch the proceedings and offer her support during her 'crying time'. These participating women were often referred to as 'gossips'—talking comforters—and this terminology is reputed to have evolved from the use by women of the herb goslip during labour.

Reports indicate that women companions kept up cheerful conversation to inspire confidence and lift the mother's spirits. They compared this birth with the others they had witnessed which were much more difficult and attempted to provoke laughter by telling bawdy jokes.

Education for birthing women and midwives

This gathering together of women for births was one way in which education took place—they learned from each other. This was particularly useful for women who wanted to gain experience so that they could assist at other births where the fee for a trained midwife could not be afforded. The observers also acted as witnesses to the birth, and this was especially relevant if the baby died. The birth and the gathering also provided an opportunity for a celebration, ably supported by the liquid refreshment available during labour.

This network of women supporting women was an early form of childbirth education—older women passing on pointers to younger ones, midwives conversing with them all. Even when men began to preside at births, it was still the midwife who was with the labouring woman throughout the 'travail'. The doctor arrived in time for the delivery only. It was also common for women who had moved away at marriage to return home for childbirth, because they preferred to be with their mothers at this time rather than with their husband's family. This suggests that an informal educational link also existed between mothers and daughters about childbirth.

Although there was no public provision for the training of early midwives, this is not to say they were regarded as untrained. A system which is based on an attitude of viewing birth as a natural process would regard a lifetime of delivering babies as more than adequate training. Some midwives followed their mothers into the profession, and others, who were of a higher class, often spent years working as an apprentice or 'deputy' with an experienced midwife before hanging the midwives' insignia—a cradle—outside their house.

This upper-class group was centred mainly in cities, and in 1690 a three-year apprenticeship in London cost a payment of five pounds to the instructing midwife. Midwifery was one of the few professions open to women who needed to earn money to support a family.

It can thus be argued that midwives held a recognised position in society and that some were well educated and well paid. Their services were also highly valued, and in pre-industrial England the female practitioner was widely trusted above her male counterpart who was well known for using blood letting as a multi-purpose treatment. Letters and diaries of the period categorically state a preference for 'midwives and old women' whose experience is rated above that of 'any physition [old English]'.

Midwives often attended the baptism or burial of infants, and their inclusion in such intimate family celebrations indicated that women's relationships with their midwives went further than 'professional' admiration. They could turn to midwives with all sorts of problems which Aristotle said, 'that they had rather die than discover to the Doctor'.

The first great woman practitioner of obstetrics, great in the sense that she both practised and trained other women and men and wrote three books on midwifery, was Louise Bourgeois. She practised at the French court and in the Hotel Dieu, the public hospital in Paris. Her midwifery text was published in 1609. She urged midwives to accept small fees and donate their services to those who could afford nothing. Her books reveal a high sense of the ethics and dignity of her profession. One of them appeared as a series of letters to 'ma fille', a daughter or a younger midwife. This is a prime example of how women passed on information to each other at this time.

Jane Sharp was the first English midwife who attempted to enlighten her professional sisters by publishing a book in 1671 on midwifery: *The Midwives' Book, or the Whole Art of Midwifery Discovered;*

Directing Childbearing Women How to Behave Themselves. She believed that midwives should improve their knowledge, particularly of anatomy, 'by a long and diligent practice', and continue to pass it on to other women.

Midwifery and witchcraft

From the fourteenth to the seventeenth centuries in Europe, England and America, the phenomenon of witchcraft and the subsequent witch-hunting dealt a serious blow to women healers and midwives. Witch-hunting began in feudal times and lasted well into the 'age of reason'.

Some feminist historians describe this witch craze as a ruling class campaign of terror directed against peasant women, who represented a political, religious and sexual threat to the church, as well as to the state. Three central accusations emerged during this time. Witches were accused of sexual crimes against men, of being organised, and of having magical powers affecting health—sometimes healing, sometimes harming. Specific charges were often levelled at obstetric skills. The *Malleus Maleficarum*, a witchhunters' manual, even stated that no one did more harm to the Catholic Church than midwives.

In performing their role as advisors on birth, contraception and abortion, midwives were bound to attract attention in such a climate. It was inevitable that the healing or pain-relieving concoctions they devised for such secret acts as sex or reproduction should be seen as evil and dangerous to the male-dominated church.

Woman's attitude to childbirth at this time was fairly matter-of-fact. It was her business and she got on with it, sometimes as the mother, other times as the helper. However, neither men nor women had full knowledge of the connection between intercourse and pregnancy, so the whole phenomenon was viewed as a somewhat super-natural happening.

Many midwives enjoyed the prestige of being possessors of 'secret skills'. Early writings tell of one midwife, Agnes Simpson, who was burned at the stake for simply having attempted to ease the labour of a woman by administering a dose of opium. Many more were charged with using 'heathen' spells and charms dictated by the devil.

There are no complete records of the number of women killed as witches. Writers vary in their estimates, but some say millions died, and they were mostly women. In a study of Essex witches, 268 of the 291 accused witches were women (92 per cent) and eleven of the men accused were either married to an accused witch or appeared in a joint indictment with a woman. Women accused of witchcraft in England and elsewhere tended to be married or widowed, to be middle-aged or old and to be of low economic status—common characteristics of midwives.

Church influence and control

During the sixteenth century, the church assumed control over the licensing of midwives in England. This action came about because the church was anxious about the popular belief in magic and the connection of the cord, caul, afterbirth and stillborn foetus with witchcraft. Under this system, the church exhorted midwives to reveal those who fell short of standards of chastity laid down by the church: they were forbidden to perform abortion; they were to press the mother to reveal the father's name so that he might support the child and be punished; and they had to baptise any child likely to die in the Anglican faith.

This 'Bishop's Licence' amounted to very little in reality. In order to obtain it, a woman had to be recommended by a few matrons, take a formal oath and pay a fee of eighteen shillings and fourpence. While this was a most effective instrument of social control, it did nothing to guarantee or improve the midwife's professional skill, as no training or examination were required.

The Judeo-Christian tradition in the West exercised a powerful influence on childbirth. Because Eve committed the original sin, women were deemed to pay forever through their own bodies according to the Bible: 'I will greatly multiply thy sorrow and thy conception; in sorrow thou shalt bring forth children; and thy desire shall be to thy husband, and he shall rule over thee.' (Genesis 3:16)

Pain in childbirth was thus seen as punishment from God and shaped men's attitude towards women negatively. Women were regarded as debased, shamed creatures, with childbirth as proof of their degraded position. Birthing women submitted to this image. They lost their intuitive approach to birth and took on expectations of fear and dread of the torturous agony of birth preached in the Bible. Earlier forms of education and healing disappeared and religious faith took precedence. As a result of these teachings, midwifery was viewed as an unclean profession and birth was seen not only as beneath the dignity of men, but also as evil incarnate.

The fear of death associated with childbirth was ever-present for women. Early tracts written specifically for lying-in women dwell on the divinely ordained hazards of childbirth and advise a hearty course of meditation of death during pregnancy. These sorts of warnings as preparation for labour no doubt led women to seek out and depend on the community of their own sex for information, companionship and assistance during birth.

Male involvement in childbirth

During the thirteenth century, with the revival of learning, the barber surgeon—a non-professional male practitioner—began to appear.

These surgeons formed a guild which undertook to train apprentices and oversee their practice. This was a much more powerful organisation than was available to midwives. Thereafter, only such trained surgeons were allowed to use the current instruments available for birth— hooks and perforators (the invention of obstetric forceps came centuries later)—and thus midwives became obliged to call upon barber-surgeons if the delivery was not straightforward. The male takeover had begun.

The witch hunts had not totally eliminated the female midwife, but she was thereafter branded as superstitious, and the way was opened for the emergence of male practitioners. Male attendants became prevalent, particularly among the middle classes, during the seventeenth and eighteenth centuries. Well before the witch hunts, male physicians had been eliminating women healers in the upper classes. By the fourteenth century, medical men had won a campaign against urban-educated women healers, and they had a clear monopoly over the practice of medicine among upper-class people. This, however, was not the case with midwifery. In all classes it remained to some extent the province of the midwife for another three centuries.

Midwives were urged not to attend women in the presence of men unless it was urgently necessary to do so. This situation arose if the delivery was complicated and the destructive instruments were needed to remove the child and save the mother. During the seventeenth century the taboo against men began to modify as the man-midwife gradually crept into the lying-in chamber. John Maubray MD, in attempting to establish his new profession, encouraged women giving birth to invite the assistance of both sexes at birth, but in his writings he clearly highlighted the superiority of men in such situations. In the eighteenth century, another factor increased male participation as it became more common for women to give birth in hospitals.

The introduction of obstetric forceps, which more than any other instrument symbolised the art of the obstetrician, as opposed to the art of midwifery, was the beginning of the end of the social, medical and educational hold of midwives over childbirth. Men gradually drove women from midwifery through the reintroduction of version and the development of the forceps. These may be described as techniques and devices which transformed the male-midwife into the saviour of dying women.

Men teaching midwives

In 1671 Jane Sharp, a midwife, saw the advent of male birth attendants as a possible threat to midwives, because of the undoubted educational advantages available to men. She pointed out the difficulties for women in acquiring good anatomical knowledge. The better trained midwives did see dissections, but they did not enjoy the same opportunities as men. Men were free to travel abroad—not possible for unattended women—and pursue their learning at universities, which were closed to women.

Moreover, the general educational opportunities open to women were greatly inferior to those offered to men. Grammar schools and universities were open only to men and the charity schools for girls aimed at fitting them for humbler occupations. The few private schools for daughters of the gentility taught needlework, fine cooking and 'accomplishments'.

Therefore, no matter how competent midwives became through experience, they were at a disadvantage, both socially and educationally, compared with men, and unlikely ever to enjoy the same prestige as them. At the close of the seventeenth century, the European tradition still required midwives to be married women of a mature age who had themselves borne children. These criteria would have ensured that midwives had domestic ties, and that they may have passed their learning peak both for new ideas and in terms of motivation. Only exceptional women like Jane Sharp were able to document their learning and the women's model of verbal exchange of information—on the job, so to speak—was totally devalued.

Attitudes towards women

In the centuries preceding antisepsis, analgesics and anaesthetic, many women must have been subjected to violent and painful deliveries if there was a complicating factor. There are publications by male practitioners with graphic descriptions of abnormal deliveries and how they were 'mastered' by the male attendant, but there is little reference to how a birthing woman coped with the insertion of a whole hand into the uterus to turn or deliver the baby, or how brutalised she might be from the insertion of blunt hooks to retrieve a dead foetus. The lack of concern by male practitioners about causing pain or mutilation to women in childbirth indicates an underlying misogyny.

Conclusion

The beginnings of the male takeover of childbirth and the struggle which ensued are part of the history of the struggle between the sexes in general and also a class struggle. Women healers and midwives were traditionally part of the people's subculture, whereas the professionals who sprung out of these times were of and for the ruling class.

These moves towards male professionalism in the childbirth area were an imposing force in the eventual development of childbirth practice amongst white Australians.

Abortion
Symbol of a world view

Jo Wainer

The abortion battle is literally about life and death. The questions it raises go to the heart of personal morality, sexual politics and the distribution of power. Each side battles to ensure space and resources for its world view. There is a 'right to life' anti-abortion movement dedicated to the preservation of the nuclear family, the primary commitment of women to child-bearing and a religious view of life which denies the value of individual choice in favour of acceptance of pain and suffering.

On the other side of the debate is the pro-choice lobby demanding that women be freed from biological destiny, that child-bearing should be a matter of choice, not chance, and expressing a secular belief that rational control of one's life is possible. The debate is not only about abortion, but also about the relationship between men and women, the resources available to women in a patriarchal society, common perceptions of female moral development and the relationship between law and morality. The abortion debate is indeed the symbol of two opposed world views.

Both anti-abortion and pro-choice groups claim to work for a more just and kind society, one which is more supportive of women and child-bearing, and rejecting of violence as a solution to personal problems. The anti-abortion, right-to-life supporters believe that outlawing abortion is a necessary step towards that kinder society, and that women must bear the cost of the long road to change. For them, abortion is early infanticide. Pro-choice supporters believe that abortion is necessary to protect women until society is more supportive of their mothering role. For them, abortion is late contraception. For one group, the women are to bear the cost of change. For the other group, the foetus is to bear the cost.

These diametrically opposed world views are founded on different economic bases. Kristin Luker has studied activists on both sides of the debate, and describes these bases as androgynous and sex-specific life resources. Androgynous life resources are created through the kinds of education, income and occupations outside the home that have been reserved for men until now. Sex-specific life resources for women are created within the 'traditional' family model: a lifetime of economic support by the husband in exchange for a lifetime of domestic labour, child-bearing and caring for children, husband and extended kin by the wife. Right-to-life people generally exist within the sex-specific model, while pro-choice people have access to androgynous resources.

Sex-specific life resources are disappearing as changing economic and social conditions reduce the 'traditional' nuclear family to a decreasing minority of family patterns. This must make those women dependent on sex-specific resources feel very threatened and accounts for some of the passion with which they fight to maintain a barrier against the tide of sexual equality. Within this model, men are restricted by the responsibility of being the breadwinner for a woman who trades domestic care for economic support. For these women sexual equality, which includes access to abortion, enables husbands to escape the restrictions and responsibilities which 'guarantee' the safety of the dependent woman.

On the other hand, nearly all pro-choice activists are women with access to androgynous resources. They too are fighting for their life. They know from experience that they cannot depend on a man to support them and they know that economic survival requires control of fertility. So arguments about who should control sexuality and reproduction are based on the crucial issues of economic, social and political control, and the focus of that control.

The second aspect of the gulf between world views is the ego-based male need to control women's sexuality and fertility. Property rights and social status passed on from father to son carry with them the need to identify, in the patriarchal society, their progeny. Access to abortion opens the possibility that women may be able to disguise the consequences of sexual activity and slip out from under the control of the male.

Most debate about abortion attempts to 'solve' the problem by answering the question, 'Is the foetus a person?' But the fact of personhood and rights of the foetus cannot be established independently of the social value foetuses and motherhood have within the culture controlling the debate.

Carol Gilligan in her book, *In A Different Voice*, points out that the construction of a context-free moral problem, 'Is the Foetus a Person?' is a characteristically male starting point. There is a difference between male and female moral development which results in different judgement and action when faced with moral dilemmas.

Referring to a number of studies which explore moral understanding and the relation between judgement and action in the lives of individuals, Gilligan asserts that women construct moral problems as problems of care and responsibility in relationships rather than as problems of rights and rules. Thus the logic underlying an ethic of care is a psychological logic of relationships which is in contrast to the formal logic of fairness that informs the characteristically male 'justice' approach.

In an abortion study described in Gilligan, women discuss the dilemmas in their lives when faced with unwanted pregnancy and the possible choices. One respondent, Claire, casts the dilemma not as a contest of rights between mother and foetus, but as a problem of relationships based on the issues of responsibility which in the end must be faced. If, because of circumstances, attachment with a baby cannot be sustained, abortion may be a better solution. Whatever the outcome, morality lies in taking responsibility for the abortion decision or taking responsibility for the care of the child. Claire's sense of connection leads her to affirm the web of relationships around her and her responsibility within that, rather than 'the sacredness of life at all costs'. Further, the abortion decision centres on the self. The concern is pragmatic and the issue is survival.

Thus the pro-life argument is based on the dominant typically male construction of morality which is context-free and characterised by a formal logic of fairness. Diametrically opposed to this world view is the typically female pro-choice position, based on a psychological morality concerned with needs and relationships.

Pro-life and pro-choice women implicitly share the understanding that the solutions to the abortion debate proposed so far do not begin to consider our fundamental needs as women. We are reduced to fighting each other in an arena circumscribed by the dominant male culture. This prevents us from joining together to reorganise social life in ways that would be constructive.

The law in Australia, and in many parts of the world, is based on the male construction of morality. Any law which requires women to give good reasons for abortion, and places the power to decide the worthiness of those reasons in the hands of a doctor or judge and jury, is treating women as though they were children, incapable of making sound moral judgements.

Women are not taken seriously when statements are made that they will have abortions for 'trivial' reasons unless regulated by the state. The most deadly anti-woman bias of all is the belief that, unless women are controlled carefully, they will pose a threat to society by killing their own progeny at random because they are not fully rational beings. Yet, as Adrienne Rich writes, women are ultimately responsible:

A man may beget a child in passion or by rape, and then disappear; he need never see or consider child or mother again. Under such circumstances, the mother faces a range of painful, socially weighted choices; abortion, suicide, abandonment of the child, infanticide, the rearing of a child branded 'illegitimate', usually in poverty, always outside the law. In some cultures she faces murder by her kinsmen. Whatever her choice, her body has undergone irreversible changes, her mind will never be the same, her future as a woman has been shaped by the event.

In his book, *Abortion: Law, Choice and Morality*, philosopher and Catholic Daniel Callahan has written:

A conviction that abortion . . . is morally wrong cannot serve as a rationale to coerce someone else with different convictions unless it can be shown that the actions . . . threaten the whole of society. It does not seem, in the instance of that form of killing we call 'induced abortion', that such a threat is present.

Anti-abortion laws coerce women throughout the world. They are the legislative expression of the dominant world view. The illegal status of abortion in many countries does not save foetuses; rather it destroys the health and takes the lives of millions of women. A review of laws and practice in a number of countries points to factors of coercion, hypocrisy and oppression of women.

The restrictive abortion laws in Cuba were changed when it was demonstrated by Professor Alvarez Lajonchere that illegal abortion was the main cause of death for women aged fifteen to 45. In other South American countries, as many as two out of three women who have self-induced or backyard abortions are admitted to hospital with injuries which threaten their life, health and reproductive capacity. Two-thirds of the beds of maternity wards in the largest women's hospital in Chile are occupied by women who have had illegal abortions. In most South American countries abortion is both illegal and a sin. The best estimate is that there is one illegal abortion for every three live births, a similar rate to that in Australia, where it is legal.

In Ireland abortion is unconstitutional, so thousands of Irish women travel to Britain each year to terminate pregnancies. In England abortion is lawful. In the United States the Supreme Court ruled in 1973 that abortion is a private matter until the foetus is viable (able to maintain an independent existence). However, in the 1989 case of *Webster vs Reproductive Health Services* the Supreme Court upheld a number of restrictions on access to abortion passed by the state of Missouri.

In Australia illegal abortion used to be a major cause of death of fertile women. Deaths from abortion are always under-reported, as they are often listed as septicaemia or haemorrhage or heart failure, rather than abortion. Despite this, in 1931 recorded abortion deaths represented 28 per cent of maternal deaths, and it was still as high as 21 per cent of maternal deaths in 1971. By the 1980s, after abortion became available legally, there were no recorded deaths from abortion until a woman died post-operatively from a ruptured ectopic pregnancy in 1984 in New South Wales.

Abortion in Australia is governed by an Act of Parliament passed in another country, in another century. The 1861 Offences Against the Person Act was passed in England and taken over by each of the Australian states in 1901. This law says that anyone who performs, or has performed upon them, an unlawful abortion, whether or not the woman was pregnant, shall be guilty of a felony. The law was passed not so much to protect the foetus, but to protect women from the very dangerous procedure that abortion once was.

The most famous Australian case was in 1969 when Dr Ken Davidson was charged with performing unlawful abortion. He pleaded not guilty, and during the trial Mr Justice Menhennitt directed the jury thus:

> For the use of an instrument with intent to procure a miscarriage to be lawful, the accused must have honestly believed on reasonable grounds that the act done by him was: (a) necessary to preserve a woman from serious danger to her life or her physical or mental health, not being merely the normal dangers of pregnancy and childbirth, which continuance of the pregnancy would entail; and (b) in the circumstances not out of proportion to the danger to be averted.

This interpretation of Section 65 of the Crimes Act is all that stands between a doctor and gaol each time she or he performs an abortion in Victoria. It clearly leaves the decision in the hands of the doctor and gives the woman no moral standing in the decision at all.

The legal position has been similar in New South Wales and Queensland. However, in 1972 a New South Wales judge directed the jury along the same lines as the Menhennit ruling, and went on to say that it was lawful to carry out an abortion in good faith if there was 'danger to mental health not only from mental disease, of disease of the mind, but from the effects of economic or social stresses'. A ruling in Queensland in 1986 confirmed the Victorian and New South Wales interpretations.

The extent to which abortion is available in Victoria indicates the ambivalent attitudes of the medical profession, and indeed the community. Abortion services are not provided in response to need, but rather are determined by staff attitudes. One of the major Melbourne hospitals determines the number of abortions it will do by constructing a ratio with live births. If we deliver X babies, we will perform Y abortions, regardless of the need. Such contempt for women. Imagine if a major public hospital were to decide that if they performed X number of tonsillectomies, they could provide Y number of kidney transplants, with no reference to need.

Abortion is now available in Victoria privately and in some public hospitals. There is one large, multi-doctor clinic and three smaller, single-doctor practices which specialise in abortion.

The two main women's hospitals, the Royal Women's and Monash Medical Centre, both have abortion services, but they have restricted access to operating-theatre time, which means many women who approach them are advised to go elsewhere. Some of the general public hospitals perform a few abortions, and most gynaecologists will terminate a pregnancy for a woman who is already their patient.

Abortion is almost unavailable in country areas, and most country women have to travel to Melbourne. Tasmanian women also come to Melbourne, as abortion is almost unobtainable in Tasmania.

Abortion is a low-status procedure in the public hospitals, and as a consequence it receives almost no funding for research or service evaluation. There is no money or research interest in the public sector for improving abortion techniques or monitoring complications. The little research being done is coming from private clinics.

The continued existence of Section 65 of the Crimes Act means that police can charge the doctor, the assisting staff and the pregnant woman with unlawful abortion every time an abortion is performed. Every abortion is potentially unlawful until proved lawful in a court of law. This has consequences for providers of abortion services, and for women who seek abortion.

It means that, perhaps subconsciously, doctors feel they are doing women a favour when they perform an abortion, and may thus feel a lesser duty to provide an excellent standard of care, to keep up with developments in the field, and to treat women with respect. Statute law and legal proceedings against doctors give the responsibility for granting or withholding an abortion to the doctor, not the woman. Some doctors respond to this by giving themselves permission to comment on the woman's morals, lifestyle and values, or by directing her on how she should be living her life.

The fact remains that doctors do continue to face a real risk of prosecution and that women who know their own minds are treated like fools.

Is there any prospect of legislative and practical change in sight? A possible factor in breaking the impasse of the abortion debate comes from the development of a medical abortifacient. This drug, known as RU 486 (Mifepristone), has been developed by the French firm, Roussel Uclef and, when taken within the first seven weeks of pregnancy, produces complete abortion in 95 per cent of women. The remaining 5 per cent require a curette to complete the abortion. Development is continuing to determine the best dosage and combination of drugs to provide complete abortion at up to eight or ten weeks' gestation.

RU 486 is being used in China and France and there is a multicentre trial being run by the World Health Organization in 23 countries throughout the world. If proven to have no dangerous side-effects, this drug could place safe abortion in the hands of general practitioners, making it much harder to stigmatise or control providers and users. There need be no record of who used it (as there is at the moment when Medicare pays the bill), and it would be up to women to take control of the medication away from doctors and into their own hands. Then abortion would truly be a private decision, carried out without interference by the state.

A resolution of the issue of abortion is not in sight. Politicians are frightened of the issue. Whatever they do, someone will hate them. There can never be community consensus and there will continue to be people with passionate commitment fighting for prohibition of abortion, or removal of legislative restrictions.

The debate on abortion will disappear from the public (as distinct from the private) arena only when there is some dramatic change in circumstances. If over-population threatens the continued survival of our society on the planet, as it does in China, then the terms of the debate may change focus. Alternatively, if a breakthrough in contraceptive technology were to permit a reversal of the norm, so that people were infertile unless they took active steps to become fertile, then the need for abortion would decrease dramatically, and so would its visibility. If abortion could become a safe chemical instead of surgical procedure, and could be removed from the control of doctors and placed in the hands of women, acting in private, then the debate would change focus. Of course, if women's ability and right to make their own decisions were recognised rather than their domination by male value systems, the situation would change.

The present conflict between anti-abortion and pro-choice forces is a fight for survival on both sides. The result is a compromise situation. Abortion may be available but possibly not legal. Women often do not have the right to decide but do anyway. The abortion debate is about power: the abortion struggle is a potent symbol of opposing world views.

References

de Beauvoir, Simone *The Second Sex* New York: Knopf, 1953

Rich, Adrienne *Of Women Born: Motherhood as Experience and Institution* New York: Norton, 1976, xiv

Callahan, Daniel *Abortion: Law, Choice and Morality* New York: Macmillan, 1970, 474

Luker, Kristin *Abortion and the Politics of Motherhood* Berkely: University of California Press 1984

Gilligan, Carol *In a Different Voice : Psychological Theory and Women's Development* Cambridge, Mass: Harvard University Press, 1982

Room to labour

The Peninsula Homebirth Support Group interviewed by Linda Martin

What made you decide to have a birth at home or think about having your next birth at home?

Jenny: I chose a home birth because I think the attitudes in hospitals are that women can't give birth without help, especially first timers. You really need to start off believing you can do it. Having my baby at home meant that I proved I could do it. And I had people at the birth who believed in me.

Kathryn: I'd like to have my own birth experience. This means that I don't want unnecessary medical interference during labour or delivery. Also so many hospital delivery rooms look like operating theatres with instruments that terrify you.

Have any of you had hospital births to compare or contrast with home birth experiences?

Jenny: My first pregnancy was a breech baby. At 37 weeks I went into hospital and delivered in the labour ward. The ward was very intimidating. I felt that I couldn't do it. Also, I went in under the threat of, 'If you don't progress, you will have a Caesarean.' I really felt I couldn't let go in the hospital—couldn't make a lot of noise. I was worried they would give me an injection of pethidine. They were talking about doing this. So there was a lot of pressure on me. Giving birth to my second child at home, I was really able to let go completely. I felt so much trust in the three people I had with me, my midwife, a girlfriend and my husband.

No one told me what to do. I was free to move, change positions, make noise, fart and do all the things that you do when you are in labour. It just didn't matter. And suddenly I delivered the head without even realising it. That's how free I felt.

When I delivered my first baby, he was whipped off. People rushed in and out cleaning up linen. There I was, strung up in stirrups, thinking, 'Leave me alone. I want my baby.'

They gave him to me for what seemed like ten seconds. I just wanted them all to go away. Everything was very official. He was a breech, and maybe he did need extra care, but he didn't need it right then.

As I said, my second child was born at home and I picked him up and discovered he was a boy. Everyone seemed to move out of my space and left me with the baby. It was actually an hour before someone said, 'I think we'd better cover him up, he's cold.' I hadn't realised that a whole hour had gone by with me just looking at my baby. No one had interfered with that. I still remember that hour as being the best time.

Jo: Our first birth was a hospital birth and we didn't know what to expect, although we had a great midwife who taught our antenatal course. She delivered our next baby at home. So with the hospital birth we were fairly well prepared. Our midwife had discussed drugs, birthing positions and being comfortable. When we arrived at the hospital we were still a little bit intimidated, but were really lucky because the midwife from the antenatal classes was on duty. So she was actually there at our birth, and it went really well.

I was in labour for ten hours. But I felt comfortable. About two hours before the baby was delivered the doctor thought I was tired, although I knew that I could have coped and gone right through. So he broke my water, and that increased the pain. The second birth was totally different. My water broke two minutes before the baby was born. I feel that would have happened in the first instance, if the doctor hadn't interfered.

Brandy: My midwife came to visit me a while after I'd had my baby at home. She told me that she had taken my chart into the hospital where she worked and showed it to a couple of doctors. She asked them whether they would have done anything differently. Both doctors said they would have broken the waters and induced the labour to make it quicker.

My labour started in the morning with very light contractions, but they were regular. It wasn't until half-past six in the evening that they started to get really exciting and things started to happen. After that it only took an hour for the delivery. The baby was born at 7.26 p.m. Obviously the doctors felt it was a long time from the morning until half-past six when nothing much seemed to be happening. They would have speeded me up a little. They are so impatient. Did they think they might fit in a few extra births or something?

Di: I was in labour for 27 hours. For the first fifteen hours it was very light. So if I had been in the hospital, I would probably have been induced. Throughout all that I was dilating very slowly. I was only five centimetres and the cervix has to dilate to eight centimetres. The baby was in a posterior position which makes for a difficult and slow labour.

If I had been in hospital, they probably would have used forceps and thus given me an episiotomy. There would also have been a chance of having a Caesarean. As it was, I didn't tear at all when I gave birth. I didn't have to worry about painful stitches around the vagina or in the stomach which may have been the case in hospital.

Also, a home birth saved me from having to make those decisions because they might have pressured me at the hospital to do so. And being very tired, I probably would have consented in the end just to get it over and done with.

Instead, I had all the support people there to help me get through it. I couldn't have done it without them. It was wonderful and I'm glad I had my baby at home.

Julie: I drew up a birth plan for the hospital which worked very well. It came about through the birth information group that I was involved with and by talking with a couple of midwives. I had to take the plan into my doctor beforehand to get it approved and signed.

At the hospital we threw the mattress on the floor. I wanted to give birth on all fours. We just started doing what we wanted. The midwife arrived, read the plan and then came over and joined our little team. It was great.

The midwife explained every stage I was going through. I was treated like an intelligent person. I was asked questions. 'Would I like this? Would I like that?'

When someone suggested that I have the injection for the placenta, I said, 'No, I'm not having it.' We just sat and talked and laughed. There I was, laughing, and the placenta arrived.

There was a surprising reaction the next day after delivery, however. They usually check to see if everything is healing up all right. No one came near me all day. Eventually a nurse on the second shift came in and said to me, 'It seems that you don't want to be touched. We've seen the birth plan and you obviously don't want to be interfered with.' I had to explain that it had nothing to do with follow-up checks.

What do people say when you tell them you are going to have your baby at home?

Julie: Things like, 'Aren't you mad? It won't be safe at home. What if something goes wrong?'

Brandy: People are fairly condescending, that's been my experience. As soon as you mention you're going to have a home birth, they think you're a little bit funny.

Kathy: Others in my family in New Zealand had had home birth experiences before, so they were very supportive. I came here and met my husband's family and they all said to me, 'If you go into labour in my house, I'm rushing you to hospital.' My husband's mother doesn't even acknowledge that I'm pregnant. She won't talk about it.

Di: My older sisters had three home births, so my parents were quite prepared for it. They were already broken in.

Jo: We told my husband's family that we were going to have our little boy present at the birth. They were really against that because they felt he wouldn't be able to cope. But he coped really well. As soon as the baby was born, he just couldn't stop looking at it and touching it. That was terrific.

Are doctors supportive of home births?

Jenny: The agreement with doctors is that if something goes wrong, the woman is transferred to hospital and the doctor will meet her there. In our area, there are no doctors who will deliver in your home.

What are your thoughts on the training and abilities of health professionals who are present at either hospital or home births?

Jenny: I think attitude counts for a lot, and being able to look at options. The current midwifery course spends the first week looking at the normal, and the final 51 weeks looking at what can go wrong. So when they get to the end of their training, there's a very distorted idea of what birth is about.

And even more so with obstetrics. When medical students are doing their obstetric training, they don't sit with a woman in labour for the whole labour and watch a normal delivery. It's like, 'Quick, there's a breech!' And they all crowd in and look at a breech, or 'We must go to theatre and see a Caesar.'

So the minute you say home birth or natural birth, a warning light goes on, and they wonder, 'What if this happens?' or 'What if that happens?' There's actually a certain number of Caesareans that have to be performed before an obstetrician can get certification. And they want to get their quota in as soon as possible.

The whole concept of birth is medicalised. You go to a doctor for your pregnancy check. You go to an obstetrician for your care. And you go to the hospital to have your baby. It really does make pregnancy seem like an illness. And on top of that there seems to be an idea that as soon as a woman becomes pregnant she's stupid.

One of the things women often say about hospital birth is that a lot of different people attend you. Nurses change shifts and other people you don't know come through.

Julie: I gave birth in a teaching hospital. I had just about everybody come in. The bed was situated right smack bang in the middle of the doorway. I was on my back with my legs up in stirrups. There was one of those screens on wheels, like a curtain, but it wasn't very high. The guys walking past were peering over the top. And I could see them doing this. Midwives came and went, so I don't really remember any particular midwife at the birth.

Brandy: People seem to forget that you're a human being. A lot of us are fairly modest about being exposed. When you're delivering you are completely exposed, emotionally and physically.

Jenny: My first delivery was a breech. During the last twenty minutes before he was born, I know that a group of onlookers came in and watched the delivery and left. They never introduced themselves and eventually disappeared without a thankyou. When I'm in labour, I'm not in a position to say anything. All I wanted was for all these people to go away. I was merely a body producing a baby.

When I was at home I had the choice of who was there. They all knew that at any time I could say, 'Please go away,' and they would, except for my midwife. But they were people I'd chosen and people that I had wanted to have there. I didn't have to worry about them and I could just get on with my labour.

Kathryn: During my first birth in a hospital, I had a series of five different midwives, none of whom bothered to speak to me. It was distancing and lonely, one of the most appalling experiences of my life.

I gave birth to my other daughter at the birth centre at the Royal Women's Hospital. She had an unusual presentation. I think it was only the second they'd had in the birth centre that hadn't been transferred out. So every single spare staff member rushed in to see the delivery. Because I'd been to prenatal classes there, I knew all their faces. They'd been supportive throughout my pregnancy and didn't impose. They were unobtrusive and interested in me as a person, not just what was happening below the waist. They maintained respect for me. I can quite understand women who only want a very small number of people around, but at that moment I didn't care. It was just so fantastic for me to know that I was actually going to push this baby out. The number of people around didn't matter.

Tell me what it was like for those of you have given birth at home.

Di: I went to the extreme. I had five support people, only because I've got some very close, wonderful friends. They wanted to be there, and I wanted them to be there. That included two guys. I actually didn't invite one of them. He just came along. It didn't bother me. He decided to go to sleep anyway, half-way through it.

As I mentioned before, I had such a long labour, 27 hours. Everybody was so tired. So when we all crashed out, this uninvited guy who had been sleeping tidied up and cooked breakfast for us when we woke up. That worked out really well. My support team was really wonderful. They were with me the whole time. They were all exhausted. They were supporting each other in the end, so I think I might have needed five of them. It was great. One of the girls, who's a photographer, took some brilliant photos.

Brandy: There's nothing nicer than giving birth at home. When Julian was born we had the stereo going. Every time I play that music the whole experience comes back to me. It really is blissful. It's so wonderful to have the baby in your own bed. You roll over and go to sleep in your own bed.

Di: I was in the bath for three hours. When I first went in it was very relaxing and it eased the contractions. After I got out, I changed positions a lot trying to get rid of the contractions but they don't go away! Some positions do relieve it a little bit though.

I was actually sitting on the toilet for a while when I had to push. That was good, because you don't have to hold your weight up as well.

In the end I actually gave birth on all fours because I was too tired to do it any other way. But it was a good position and I liked it. I was leaning over my husband.

Jo: Our midwife brought a birthing stool to our house. For the first hour of labour, I sat on it. The birthing stool was very comfortable. But I didn't even think of it during the actual birth. I was planning to have a bath, and I didn't get a bath. I was planning to have a tape recording of the baby's heartbeat but I didn't get that either. The birth happened so quickly, I didn't have time to do anything.

Jenny: My support people had this big list of questions. 'Would you like to take a walk? Would you like to dance? Do you want to change positions?' I had all sorts of ideas for different positions. But when the actual time comes you just follow your instinct.

What happened right after your babies were born?

Kathryn: In both my birth experiences I held my babies right from the beginning and didn't let go for hours. I was persistent in hospital and they didn't argue with me. That was fine. In the birth centre it was expected that you would hold your baby right away, so I wasn't under any pressure. I fed my baby immediately. That was terrific. I knew it was a very important time for me, because my labour had been so ghastly and the birth experience so appalling. I had to reclaim my child. That bonding time is so important. I overindulged myself in it, to the extent that my husband was also a little bit jealous for a while.

Some women say that one of the positive things about giving birth in hospital is you get a chance to rest. How do you manage after a home birth?

Jenny: My husband was home for a week and a half after my second child was born so he was able to help out. I had a freezer full of food. I had a heap of really good friends who came and did my housework, my shopping, or took my toddler away if I needed it. So I got as much rest as I wanted. I was awake when the baby was awake.

But I think it's really important to set yourself up beforehand. So if people offer to help you, accept it. In fact, I had more sleep than I did in hospital, because hospitals have routines. If your baby's been awake all night and you've just gone to sleep at six in the morning, and the routine starts at six, they wake you up again.

Did any of you think about what might happen if there was an emergency during your home birth?

Brandy: Everybody tried to tell me to think about it. I had to be booked in at the hospital just in case. But no matter how negative people were, I was optimistic that nothing would go wrong.

Di: I thought about it, but not at the birth. I spoke about it with my midwife earlier. I trust her totally. She continually monitors you through the whole birth. She actually monitors you more at home than she does when she's working in the hospital. So you're even more closely watched by her than you would be if you were in hospital. She also has you booked into the hospital. You make arrangements with the obstetrician. If there is any problem the midwife contacts him and we all meet at the hospital. So it's all pretty well covered. I felt totally confident.

Jenny: All possibilities are actually covered. If there are any problems during the pregnancy our midwife has the responsibility of telling us that we are not suitable for home birth. If something goes wrong during labour or delivery we trust the midwife to tell us, 'It's time to go to the hospital.' My midwife brings a whole range of resuscitation equipment for baby and mother.

Di: When my baby was born, my midwife looked at the placenta and said, 'My God, look at this!' What had happened was the cord had actually grown through the membrane before it joined to the placenta. So when my waters broke, the possibility of breaking the cord was there. And the membrane broke not far from where the cord was. If that had happened, no matter what sort of monitoring, whether in hospital or at home, the baby would have died instantly through loss of blood. The midwife had seen three of those in her ten years of practice. The other two were in hospital, and one of those babies died. So there is no guarantee either at home or in hospital on how safe a birth will be.

How was this homebirth support group formed and what have you derived from it?

Jenny: I started off the group after I had my baby at home, because I found while I was pregnant I really needed support from other people, to tell me that my choice was 'OK. I knew it was, but it's really hard to have criticism thrown at you quite consistently.

So after he was born, I wrote a letter to half a dozen people I knew who had had births at home. They all came to my house one morning for a cup of coffee. I threw out some ideas and everyone thought they were great. So it took off from there. Our group has been going for about seven months. We meet every six weeks and I write a quarterly newsletter to keep people in touch. The meetings are generally social. We try to make new people welcome. It's a chance for women to come and hear other stories and get a bit of positive reinforcement. We've all made some really great friends through this group.

Julie: This group is useful because it includes women who have already given birth and those who are about to give birth. When I was in the birth information group before this, women didn't come back after they delivered. With this group I can pass on my experience and knowledge to other women.

Jo: I found support through this group. I didn't have anyone to talk to about having a home birth, so it was great to get together with women who had been through it. There was no negativity. People weren't saying, 'What if . . . ?'

Enough is enough
Women's experiences of In Vitro Fertilisation

Renate Klein

Increasingly, the new reproductive technologies, especially in vitro fertilisation (IVF), are being exposed as ineffective, often health-endangering and dehumanising technologies which seldom provide infertile people with their much-desired child, but on the contrary use living women as experimental test-sites for drugs, new technological procedures and suppliers of 'raw material'—eggs and embryos for experimentation.

Feminists all over the world are alerting the public to the fact that these technologies are a further stepping-stone in the patriarchal quest to conquer that last grand scientific frontier: the production of children by taking control of the process of baby-making. In addition to these analyses, I believe it is crucial that women who have been on test-tube baby programs talk about their own experiences and make them public. What do they think, feel and experience in their journey from longing for a biological child, through encountering difficulties in conceiving, to eventually undergoing IVF? How do technological interventions influence their physical and emotional well-being, their sense of self? Do they feel in control of the IVF process? Are they informed of health hazards, of documented deaths? Above all, have they been told that IVF remains an experimental procedure? Finally, how do the 95 per cent of women who quit the IVF program without a child cope?

Methods used in the study
These were the questions that prompted me to undertake an exploratory survey of 40 Australian women who had undergone IVF and left it without a child. I wanted to hear women speak for themselves about their experiences with reproductive medicine.

Critics might say that my study does not encompass women who were satisfied with their experience of IVF, despite the fact that it was not successful. I believe strongly that the reverse is true: that there is a bias in my survey towards women who felt they *could* cope with their past IVF experience, who *were* emotionally capable of writing and talking about it.

Almost without exception, the women in my study are well educated and middle-class, and had strong support from their partners. In other words I would argue that the often harsh words spoken by respondents in my survey reveal only the tip of the iceberg of what women have to go through in their IVF experience. Women whose lives were wrecked by the trauma of being 'living laboratories' at the hands of some particularly ruthless, success-oriented and misogynist doctors and scientists did *not* reply to the advertisements I placed in the main Melbourne papers for respondents for my study.

The women in my report are speaking about 'the other side' of IVF, the side not written about in the glossy magazines.

The women's experiences

The majority of the 40 women in my study were between 30 and 35 years old with slightly older partners. (Three women were under twenty and five over 40.) All but two were married. Prior to going on IVF, 35 were in paid employment; however, at the time of my study (two to six months after leaving IVF), only 26 were employed: a marked drop.

Roughly half the women had been involved in the IVF program for two years; for most of the remainder, it was three or four years. Most commonly, a woman made three attempts, while several tried as many as five times; only one woman only tried once. The total number of attempted IVF cycles in my study was 126 between the 40 women.

The costs were significant: thirteen women paid between $3000 and $4000, seven between $5000 and $6000, five over $6000 and three under $2000. (The other women seemed to have blocked out how much they had actually spent on IVF; one spoke for many when she said, 'So much, you don't even want to think about it'.) The majority said they were refunded roughly half the cost.

The women's experiences leave no doubt that infertility can be a shattering experience. As one woman put it: 'I felt emotionally distraught, worthless, extremely upset, and angry. It was bitter disappointment, social rejection—a feeling of being incomplete.'

Once the women had taken steps to find out why they did not become pregnant and saw a doctor, the majority of them—35—only told family and close friends, afraid of the serious stigma attached to infertility with blame often being placed on the infertile woman. Thus many women saw no other way to deal with the problem than to pursue endless years of pain and trauma, first in conventional infertility treatments, later in IVF.

Many felt they had become outcasts in their own families. As one woman put it: 'Increasingly, I felt displaced at family events. Everyone had children but us. And although I'd just been promoted I know Mum's eyes would have lighted up much more if I had announced "I'm pregnant".' Due to such problems, 30 women in my study seemed to have internalised the fertility problem and felt guilty about it, even women in couples where it was the male who was infertile.

As many as 32 women said that the issue of infertility took a heavy toll on their relationship. Twelve felt that in the end the infertility problem had strengthened it, but that, when undergoing the various treatments, it had been very stressful. As one woman summarised: 'It caused a lot of tension; we faced enormous emotional problems and had to decide if we would remain together as a couple.'

Altogether, then, many of the women in my study experienced infertility as a serious life crisis. As society, in which a 'proper' woman is still defined as a mother, tends implicitly to stigmatise the childless woman, many women's self-esteem and well-being are seriously affected by the verdict 'infertile'. Many told me that their whole sense of self became shaky; they experienced 'a feeling of being displaced', 'of not belonging'.

Commencing IVF: Most women had had a long, painful and disappointing history of unsuccessful medical interventions in the quest for fertility. For them, IVF appeared to be 'the last opportunity open to us'. Although 35 of the 40 women in my study did see problems with IVF (the most frequent of which was that they felt unsure whether they would be able to cope emotionally), one spoke for many when she said: 'A chance was better than none; at least we could say that we'd tried the latest technology.'

Some women who sought information on the nature of the treatment and the demands put on them felt very frustrated that they weren't told what the IVF procedure really entailed: 'Information was scarce. The first time was filled with excitement at the possibilities. Talks with the medical practitioners were brief purely because there was never an answer to our particular problem. "Everyone" was always guessing at possible solutions.' Another woman commented: 'I felt like a Friesian cow ready to be experimented upon. I did not feel like a person after talking to Professor X. The team aren't interested in people, only in science.'

There are serious health risks to women from the IVF procedure, particularly from overstimulation of the ovaries to get more than one mature egg or from accidents during egg collection. There may also be risks to their children from IVF drugs. I wanted to know whether there had been discussion of these potential dangers in the initial stages of IVF. Alarmingly, of the 40 women, only nine said there had been such discussions. Morever, if 'side-effects' were mentioned at all, advice ranged from, 'Not a great deal of side-effects' (one), 'dizziness/nausea' (two), 'weight increase' (one), 'Hormone levels will be affected' (one), 'Lots of eggs will be produced' (one), 'Multiple births possible' (two). One woman was told 'not to worry'. Only one woman out of the 40 was given an answer regarding long-term effects: 'It's a new science . . . we are not aware of potential long-term side effects.'

In my view, conducting human experiments without even informing the research 'subjects' that they are part of an ongoing experiment rather than a 'routine' safe procedure is, quite plainly, medical malpractice. It also exploits a particularly vulnerable group of people. As one woman put it: 'I was worried about the lack of information. I knew we were guinea pigs but I could not find any literature. Also, I desperately wanted IVF to work . . . and to believe the doctors who told me not to worry.'

The IVF procedure: Reports from the women in my study, on their reactions to the drugs they took when on the IVF program, confirmed the health hazards reported in the international research literature. Thus almost half the women in my study (nineteen) mentioned adverse effects from the superovulation treatments, specifically with the fertility drug clomiphene citrate, marketed frequently as Clomid. Nine reported the development of cysts which meant that the IVF treatment had to be stopped. (*Note:* For a detailed discussion on clomiphene citrate and 'hormonal cocktails' given in conventional infertility treatment and IVF, see Klein/Rowland [1988] and Klein [1989].)

Alarmingly, this study also confirms that Australian doctors, like their peers who publish in the international research literature, do not always adhere to the maximum dosages recommended by the drug manufacturer. In the case of Clomid, MIMS, the directory of medical and pharmaceutical products, recommends 50 mg for five days and says that if ovulation but not pregnancy occurs, two additional cycles of 100 mg for five days 'up to a total maximum of six cycles of Clomid treatment may be administered'. Yet in my survey, four women were on 150 mg daily, and one was on 50 mg for an entire year. Another woman recalled:

I started with one tablet a day but when the ultrasound revealed that my eggs did not grow properly I was told to increase the dosage up to four tablets [200 mg] a day. Then I was 'cancelled'.

My ovary had swollen considerably and despite attempts to release ripe follicles, no mature eggs were recovered.

There are, however, worrying indications that in fact there is no such thing as a 'safe' dose of clomiphene citrate. One woman who was on a low dosage (i.e. 50 mg for three days) developed a cyst and had to stop the IVF treatment. Another woman who had been given 50 mg for five days wrote to me:

My third attempt: sixteen eggs good size; when pick-up happened found cyst, lost eggs. No success. I was told my cyst had killed off my eggs but when I was unclear they told me they had drained my cyst and I could come in on my next cycle. After going home and having much pain I went back to my own doctor and was told I would have to go into hospital and have the large cyst removed. I could also lose one or both of my ovaries. I was very upset with this as it meant ten days in hospital, six weeks off work, and my fourth long operation. If I had taken my IVF doctor's advice who can say what would have happened.

These kinds of gruesome experiences unfortunately continued in the second stage of the program, egg pick-up. One woman told me that following egg collection by laparoscopy, she had a high fever and ended up in intensive care with a severe infection: she could have died. Another woman, despite a heavy dose of antibiotics provided as a preventative measure after egg pick-up via the vagina, also developed a serious infection. This inflamed her tubes and provided great cause for concern that she might have been rendered infertile by the IVF procedure: she was on the program because of her husband's infertility.

Mixed with these stories of actual bodily harm come tales of extreme tension, anxiety and stress. Asked whether she felt any side-effects from the drugs administered, one woman said:

It became a battle even doing part-time work. I could never let them know exactly when I was going into hospital and they naturally resented this. I felt that they would have preferred my resignation, but I didn't feel I could give up work even though my doctor had suggested this. But I thought, if I give up work and don't have a baby, then what will I have? What would I do with my time?

Many women felt during this time that they were 'just machines', guinea pigs 'on the assembly line', as one woman called the IVF program. Many commented that doctors did not place a great deal of importance on them as human beings: 'for them you are just X, just another number'. One woman said: 'I felt like a baby machine; no one was interested in me as a person. I was just a chook with growing eggs inside—and if they didn't grow properly then it was my own fault.'

More than two-thirds of the women who had reached the egg pick-up stage in at least one of their attempts, (34 women with a total of 75 attempted cycles at this stage) said they experienced some after-effects from this procedure. For fourteen it was feeling nauseous and dizzy from the anaesthetic after a laparoscopy; seven others complained of abdominal discomfort; seven got infections. For some this was the final blow: they decided to stop. As one woman put it, 'enough is enough'.

> Following the third ovum pick-up the gynaecologist told me my tubes were OK but my ovaries were bound by adhesions which prevented him from collecting the numbers of eggs which were there. He advised microsurgery via laparoscopy which would increase my chances of a pregnancy and allow more access to my ovaries if a further pick-up was to be done. However, I developed an ovarian abscess and infection which necessitated three weeks in hospital—two further operations and removal of one ovary and tube, and four different types of intravenous antibiotics. When I recovered, I realised my health and time with my husband was far more important than an endless endeavour to conceive a baby. At this stage, too, we were awaiting approval from the Welfare Department to adopt a child.

For the women who continued their IVF cycles (between one and eight attempts), the wait now began: waiting to hear whether the eggs had been fertilised. This period was experienced by many 'as feeling totally out of control'. Six women complained that their eggs were 'lost' or 'mixed up' or, as one woman was told, 'cooked'. There was also general dissatisfaction with the explanations given to them:

> It was my third attempt and they got ten eggs from me. They put four embryos back but I don't know what happened to the other six. They wouldn't really give us a proper explanation. They just said they were either immature or they weren't dividing properly or something like that. You really don't know what's happened to them.

When there was no fertilisation, this particular IVF attempt had come to an end. This was the case eighteen times. As well as these, there were other problems: on two occasions the partner could not produce sperm, in another six instances there was something 'wrong' with the sperm; in another five there was something 'wrong' with the eggs. (When frozen embryos were being used, in ten cases these did not thaw out undamaged.) One woman remembers the painful experience:

> When I was told that my eggs weren't good enough and that I should give up I was shocked and utterly devastated. I remained deeply depressed for more than a year and I was suicidal a lot of the time. I felt such an abysmal failure, a barren woman unable to give my husband a child and my parents their grandchildren. I had even failed technology.

The next hurdle was the embryo transfer. The procedure itself, was declared 'manageable' by all but one of the women. Nevertheless, it was described as 'embarrassing' and 'humiliating' by eight women: lying in stirrups, head down, legs up and having the product of conception—your future baby—inserted through your cervix is indeed the epitome of powerlessness and vulnerability. One woman recalls a particularly enraging experience:

> I remember the first embryo transfer I had. At the time there were visiting doctors from IVF programs around the world, and I happened to be one of the guinea pigs going in for the transfer on the day they were at the hospital. It is embarrassing enough lying there with your legs up in stirrups without a roomful of people staring at you and with a huge spotlight [theatre light] shining on your genitals! When my doctor said to me that after that day I would have an 'international fanny' I was really annoyed at this remark, and the innuendo that I should somehow be thrilled at the prospect of being seen by all these international doctors.

After the embryo transfer came the stressful time of waiting to see if the pregnancy had started or, in the medical jargon, if the embryo had 'taken'. All the women who had made it to this point at least once in their IVF history felt that this was the most trying time of the whole procedure. One echoed the sentiments of many when she said: 'I could hardly stand it. I didn't feel I knew what to do—every move seemed dangerous; when driving, after every little bump I was convinced: that was it—I've lost it.' But, as confirmed in the literature, the embryo transfer is the stage in the IVF procedure when two out of three attempts come to an end. Indeed, out of 30 women with a total of 88 embryo transfers between them, only six women got beyond this point. For three of those, their pregnancies ended with an early miscarriage and for the other three with an ectopic pregnancy. So of the 40 women who had, between them, attempted IVF 126 times, none had a child in the end.

Most women said that finding out that an embryo transfer had not worked was the hardest part of the process. One woman said: 'I can't describe the feelings accurately but I think it is akin to being grief stricken. Also the feeling of, "Oh God, I've got to go through all this again in the next cycle." It is utter despair and extreme isolation. You feel you are a dismal failure.'

The time after IVF: Asked what made them finally decide not to try again, nineteen women said, 'I couldn't cope with the emotional stress any more.' One woman commented, 'I couldn't face the ups and downs', and eight noted, 'I couldn't bear the uncertainty.' As one woman said: 'Each time there was anticipated hope followed by devastation, crying, emotional upset. After the third attempt, I felt that I could not go through with all the emotional strain any more.'

Physical risks were mentioned too: 'risks of infection' (six); 'wanted to withdraw from drugs' (five); 'surgery *because* of IVF was too much' (three); 'miscarriage' (one); as well as problems with the partner because, 'our future was up in the air' (fourteen); 'stress on sex life' (eight); 'his inability to cope with my misery while on the program' (three); 'his inability to cope with negative results' (two).

Financial problems also influenced the decision to stop. 'It took all my wages', said four women. So did problems at work: 'I ran out of sick leave' (six); 'I couldn't juggle work and IVF any more' (nine).

Four women stated that they left because they had stopped believing in IVF. As one put it, 'I lost all trust in IVF.' Fifteen women specifically mentioned the negative role the IVF doctor(s) played and how totally disempowered they felt. As one put it:

> When I first came with my list of questions, Dr X patted me on my head and said, 'Now don't you worry your little head off. We know what's best for you, so if you co-operate and stop worrying, you'll have a good chance.' Later, however, he stopped being so 'nice' and once, when I complained about his assistant being too late for egg pick-up . . . he commented sharply, 'Doctors' wives always cause trouble', and 'You want a child, don't you? If you do, then give up your job, stop being a problem and co-operate.' So I felt I had to shut up or risk delay on the program.

Eventually, however, she could not take it any longer: 'I felt I was reduced to a pin cushion test case; it began to erode my sense of identity.' Four other women said that gradually, while still on the IVF program, they began to accept infertility as a part of their lives which helped them to stop. As one put it: 'Each day I woke up and said to myself, "There is more to life than IVF. I must accept that we won't have our own child."'

Once the decision was made to leave IVF behind, the women were left totally to their own devices. Many women complained that there were no services available to cope with the feelings of desperation, let-down, anger, and—perhaps worst—in many cases not knowing what to do next. Only two were offered counselling. As one said angrily:

> They courted me because I seemed an 'interesting case'. But when it hadn't worked three times—and I had asked too many questions—I was dropped like a hot potato. No one was interested in me any more; in fact they clearly wanted to get rid of me. Somehow I must have reminded them of their failure . . . I was a bad statistic.

This lack of support and counselling at the end of IVF is scandalous. It is one indication that IVF is indeed not about helping and supporting infertile people, but rather about control over the process of baby-making. If a woman delivers 'bad' goods, that is, she doesn't even get pregnant, she is thrown by the wayside and a fresh one, a promising case, takes her place.

Just as important as the production of babies is the access to embryos which the IVF procedure makes possible. By experimenting on embryos and developing a multitude of tests to screen embryos— with the intent to eliminate those 'unfit' to be born by not implanting them in the woman's womb—the application of IVF is extending to a rapidly growing number of people. Indeed it is already being advocated as the future method of procreation for all people: a deeply alarming prospect as it would mean further control over which women in which countries are allowed to produce what kind of children— and who decides!

Conclusions

The IVF story as told by the majority of women for whom IVF does not work bears little resemblance to the fairytales we read in glossy magazines. It is a story of pain, emotional distress and ill health—and no baby at the end. It is also one of disturbing medical malpractice in which the emotional vulnerability of a group of women is badly abused: they are literally 'vivisected' as they become living test-sites. As a consequence, the women may suffer serious long-term ill-health, disturbed hormonal cycles, perhaps early menopause or maybe worse (i.e. cancer). Even the few children who are born from IVF may have health problems when they reach adulthood— for example, fertility problems and increased incidence of cancer.

The human factor in IVF—played up by IVF practitioners to gain public acceptance—is strongly disputed by the participants in this study. The women were almost unanimous in their verdict of the doctors. With very few exceptions they were described as 'cold', 'up themselves', 'only interested in science, not people'. The comments on the absence of meaningful counselling, particularly after IVF, were equally damning. In sum, then, as one woman said: 'The only ones it works for are the doctors and scientists—not us!'

This study has confirmed that IVF is not in women's best interests: it seldom produces babies, it often makes women ill and seriously destabilises their whole sense of self and, in fact, it is a new form of violence against women. This is why IVF—a failed and dangerous technology—must be stopped.

References

Bachman, Christian 'Vom Sinn der Unfruchtbarkeit and vom Stress der Bermachtig Ersehnten Kinder' *Tages-Anzeiger Magazin*, (Zurich, Switzerland), no. 9, 28 February 1987, 16–23

Klein Renate *Where Choice Amounts to Coercion: The Experiences of Women on IVF Programmes* paper presented at 3rd Interdisciplinary Congress on Women, Dublin, Ireland, 6–10 July 1987

—— 'When Medicalisation Equals Experimentation and Creates Illness: The Impact of New Reproductive Technologies on Women' *Sortir la Maternité du Laboratoire* Gouvernement du Quebec, 1987

—— *The Exploitation of a Desire: Women's Experiences with In Vitro Fertilisation* Geelong, Vic.: Deakin University Press, 1989

—— (ed.) *Infertility: Women Speak Out About Their Experiences of Reproductive Medicine* London: Pandora Press and Sydney: Allen & Unwin, 1989

—— 'Resistance: From the Exploitation of Infertility to an Exploration of Infertility' in Renate D. Klein (ed.) *Infertility: Women Speak Out* London: Pandora Press and Sydney: Allen & Unwin, 1989

Klein, Renate and Rowland, Robyn 'Women as Test-Sites for Fertility Drugs: Clomiphene Citrate and Hormonal Cocktails' *Reproductive and Genetic Engineering: Journal of International Feminist Analysis* 1, 3, 1988, 251–73

MIMS Annual, 1987 Crows Nest, NSW: IMS Publishing, 1988

Rowland, Robyn 'Reproductive Technologies: The Final Solution to the Woman Question?' in Rita Arditti, Renate Klein and Shelley Minden (eds) *Test-Tube Women: What Future for Motherhood?* London: Pandora Press, 365–70

Stanley, Fiona 'In Vitro Fertilization—a Gift for the Infertile or a Cycle of Despair?' *Medical Journal of Australia* 148, 2 May 1988, 15–19

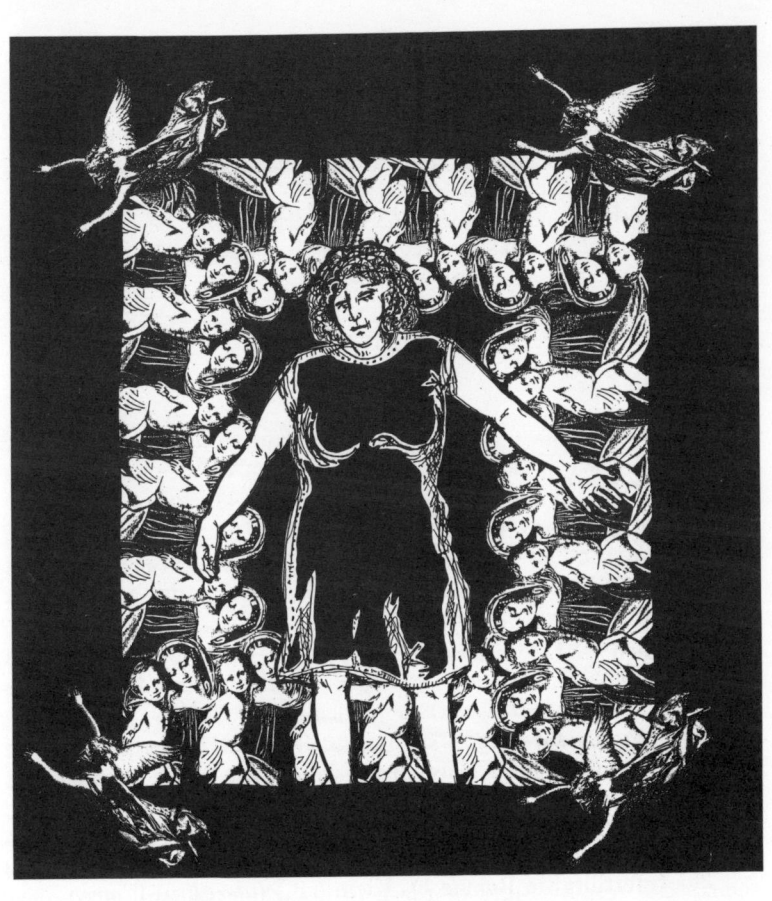

Motherhood, Deborah Kelly, 1986

IVF

The package deal

Robyn Rowland[1]

In spite of the rhetoric of compassion constantly pushed at the public
by medical researchers in the new reproductive technologies, it is
clear that IVF (in vitro fertilisation) scientists and practitioners are
not benign prophets of the future. Rather they are involved in
increasing masculine control over reproduction and procreation, and
in developing businesses which have the primary aim of making a
profit from the needs of infertile people.

In this paper, I will describe briefly the social context in which
these technologies are being developed, bearing in mind that we are
discussing here social rather than medical issues.

There are several aspects of the social environment which need
our attention. First is what has been termed 'masculine' science, and
its associated values of controlling, dominating and exploitating nature,
rather than co-operating with it.[2] Scientists frequently show themselves to be capable of only a narrow tunnel-vision, refusing to accept
their social responsibility or the controls which society endeavours
to place upon them. This masculine control is evident in the history
of the relationship between women and medicine. Here the issue of
control has been played out historically and continues today. Not
satisfied with the natural ovulation of a woman, IVF practitioners
endeavour to control her cycle, then superovulate her 'under control'[3]
by giving her drugs to make her ovaries produce more than the normal
one egg per cycle.

Even more horrifying is the fact that women are constantly used
as experimental subjects in medical trials or research. One example
of this was the use of DES (diethylstilboestrol), a synthetic oestrogen.
This drug was used from the early 1940s until 1971 as a drug for
pregnant women prone to miscarriage. Some women taking the drug
were told by their doctors that they were taking vitamins. But DES
had a 'time-bomb' effect: years later daughters of these women have
increased risks of cancer of the vagina.

As well, these women experienced higher rates of infertility, spontaneous abortion, ectopic pregnancy and premature delivery. Sterility problems have been detected in some of the sons of DES mothers. And, more than 30 years after they used the drug, the women who took DES are suffering breast cancer rates which are 40 to 50 per cent higher than other women their own age.[4]

Surely it is extraordinary that IVF is now hailed as a solution to the problems of DES. DES daughters are being offered IVF pregnancies to overcome their infertility caused by medical mismanagement and experimentation on their mothers.[5]

Medical experimentation on women still continues. An appalling example was recently uncovered—a 30-year experiment on women at Auckland's National Women's Hospital. In this study, which should have been stopped by the hospital's ethics committee, women who had cancer *in situ* were used as a control group, being denied treatment for purposes of comparison with another group. Unknowingly, they became living research experiments as doctors routinely checked them and documented the 'progress' of their cancerous cells, failing to intervene even to save their lives. Twelve women have died as a result. If it had not been for the work of two feminist health activists, Phillida Bunkle and Sandra Coney, and their book, *The Unfortunate Experiment*, this use of women as guinea pigs would never have become public. The superintendent-in-chief of the hospital board refused to follow up several complaints by doctors over the twenty years of this experiment, claiming that there was 'insufficient evidence' to take action, despite documentation which included accounts of the deaths of two women.[6]

A second element in the social context is the manner in which reproductive technology is dismembering and fragmenting women. Using what I would term 'Reprospeak' researchers depersonalise women, who are described merely as wombs, eggs, ovaries—body parts disconnected from the women and their lives. So Dr Robert Winston, a British IVF scientist, describes surrogate mothers as 'endocrinological environments'; Judge Harvey Sorkow, who heard the Mary Beth Whitehead case, described surrogates as 'alternative reproduction vehicles'; and the American Fertility Society described them as 'therapeutic modalities'.[7]

Eggs and embryos take on lives of their own, becoming personalised at the expense of women. They can be 'orphaned' or 'parentless' (as in the case of the Rios embryos) and of 'good quality' or 'poor quality'. They may even be 'wayward' if they don't stay where the doctors put them.[8]

Scientists using 'Reprospeak' try to 'soften up' the public. So Dr Yovich in Perth can suggest that the problematic issue of multiple births on IVF programs means that the programs are 'too effective';[9] the failure rates of IVF become 'success rates'; and the death of a Perth woman on an IVF program becomes a 'therapeutic misadventure' in the words of the coroner and is described by Dr Alan Trounson as a 'terrible side effect'.[10]

Women's bodies have traditionally been treated by the medical profession as defective machines in need of improvement and control. Discussing the possible relationship between ovulation and development of ovarian cancer, Dr Fathalla writes in the English medical journal, *The Lancet*: 'Compared with other mammals . . . Women have extravagant and mostly purposeless ovulation'.[11] So ovarian tumours are caused because women are just far too lavish with their eggs. And use of the term 'purposeless' suggests that ovulation may not be well understood by science and medicine!

Women's bodies are stubborn even *after* medical intervention! Discussing chromosomal errors as the reason for a loss of embryos in IVF, Alan Trounson writes that 'it is plausible that some of these chromosomal errors may result in the *failure* of the *mother* to respond to the presence of the embryo'.[12]

Losing their identity and personality, women are also seen by researchers as research animals. Again Drs John McBain and Alan Trounson write, 'the human female is capable of having substantial litters . . . '.[13]

A third element in the social context of reproductive technology is the relationship between commerce and medical science. There are many financial institutions whose profit is rooted in women's bodies. These include the reproductive 'supermarkets' in North America, the drug and pharmaceutical companies, and commercial companies specifically established to sell reproductive technology and genetic engineering.

Apart from the massive investment in genetic engineering, reproductive technology profit comes largely through operating clinics and the infertility drug pharmaceutical market. In Australia three main companies have, since November 1988, been established to make a profit from infertility or to generate research funds: IVF Australia (IVFA) (since November 1988, Australian Medical Investments), Pivet in Perth, and the Infertility Medical Centre in Melbourne. IVFA has established North American clinics in Rochester, New York and Birmingham, Alabama. Both these clinics have announced they are intending to expand into regional areas. Some companies operate on venture capital and others have floated public stock issues. The public issue for CP Ventures which established IVF Australia was underwritten in part by the Victorian Economic Development Corporation (state owned).[14] In 1988 IVFA was looking to establish clinics in Singapore, Japan and other countries. The profit forecast is $6.5 million for each clinic per year in revenue when they are fully operational.[15]

The Perth company Pivet (Programmed In Vitro Fertilisation and Embryo Transfer) has been established to 'tap potential multi-billion dollar untouched markets in Britain, Europe, Asia, North Africa and the Middle East'. It is selling scientific know-how, equipment and computer software. In a quaint discussion of funds, it is indicated that Western Australia's IVF program began from a modest beginning from 'funds raised through lamington drives and the sale of home-made jams and cakes by a loyal and dedicated band of childless wives and would-be grandmothers'. Pivet Australia has developed into a $5 million complex with a team of scientists and technicians of inter-national reputation. In 1988 it established a laboratory in Pantai, Malaysia and in 1986 set up a similar complex in Kuala Lumpur—the Subang Medical Centre. A further complex has been established in Athens and other laboratories are planned for Hong Kong, Naples, Singapore, Cairo and Britain. Infertility treatment and equipment is a lucrative export commodity.[16]

There are many more issues associated with this commercialisation than there is space to explore here, including the threat to academic freedom and the possibility of the abuse of women in the drive for profits. But, importantly, we must note that, although medical scientists and practitioners give us the 'soft sell' on their concern for infertile couples, the reality is that infertility treatment is big business.

The second important point is that, because of the relationship now developed between commercial enterprises and medicine, it does not pay medicine to cure infertility. Companies need a continuing infertile population. As Blakeslee comments, 'To be profitable, IVF clinics must generate high patient volume to cover the extremely high fixed and operating costs associated with IVF'.[17]

To this end, Vicki Baldwin of IVF Australia has said 'we invest heavily in public relations'.[18] As Dr John Kerin of the University of Adelaide's Queen Elizabeth Hospital said before he left to take up a new position in the United States: 'there is more than enough for everyone'.[19] And finally, Dr Glick, president of the Genex Cor-poration said: 'I do not know how to emphasise this too much but it is the stock incentive that has really turned the scientists on. I think there is a lesson to be learned here.' Indeed!

There is even an Australian IVF tourist package for Japanese would-be parents! They will stay at the Allamanda Private Hospital in Southport which claims 'Australia's highest success rates for test-tube babies'—after 35 *pregnancies*, not live births. The clinic is overseen by Professor Carl Wood from Melbourne. Services are being offered to Japanese, New Zealand, Filipino and Singapore couples—at a price.[20]

The fourth aspect in the context behind reproductive technology is social attitudes to infertility and particularly to mothering. Living in a society which defines people who have children as 'good' pressure is placed constantly on people, but particularly women, to create families. Having a child supposedly marks a status passage from childhood to maturity and defines women as whole beings.

With this kind of attitudinal background, women experience infertility as a painful life crisis. Most importantly, it marks for people a sense of loss of control over something which we all assume we do control. It is that sense of control which many infertile people hope to regain through their involvement in IVF and associated programs. Studies carried out with women on IVF programs, however, indicate that, on the contrary, they feel used as laboratory animals or, as women themselves describe it, as a 'Friesian cow', 'a hamster on a wheel', 'as guinea pigs'.[21]

The fifth factor in the social context of IVF is the considerable cost to individual couples. But so too is the cost to the Australian community through government funding of health services. In 1987, the estimated total costs of IVF alone to the Australian government was $30 million. The report estimates that the average cost of each live baby is about $40 500 with a cost to government of $22 680.[22]

But these costs do not include the previous infertility treatment, nor obstetric and perinatal costs. Although some costs to patients are not legitimately part of Medicare, accounting devices can be used to change the billing for procedures which do not have a Medicare number to procedures which do have a number.[23] In addition, patients, instead of paying for laboratory processes, often make a tax deductible 'donation' to the research program which means that they can recoup a significant part of their expenses through the taxation system.

The community pays through the hospitalisation and expensive neonatal care needed, through the use of hospital facilities and expertise, through a general use of a limited health budget—and all for a technology that is basically a failure. This occurs at a time in Australia when Aboriginal children are dying from something as simple as diarrhoea because they do not get adequately financed health care.

It is interesting to examine the medical research budget from the National Health and Medical Research Council for 1988 to consider levels of government expenditure on IVF-related research in comparison with allocations to areas that directly affect women's health. Genetically related research received almost $2 million, IVF-related research received $433 913, while no money was given to the prevention of infertility. In comparison, community health research was allocated $160 000, and one of the greatest killers of women, breast cancer, received a mere $42 923.[24]

As a community we have to ask: are such costs acceptable when they amount to paying science to experiment on women with the intention of developing greater profits for themselves? The Australian government report notes:

> IVF is a new procedure, involving new technology. It is high cost and discretionary. In addition there are questions about the success of the procedure, the long term safety of some drugs used in IVF and the high rate of congenital malformations and low birth weight infants among IVF children. Under other circumstances, a new procedure such as this would be subject to assessment and evaluation before such high levels of Commonwealth funds were committed.[25]

The use of the drug Clomid (clomiphene citrate) to stimulate ovulation is of particular concern. Side-effects include complaints such as dizziness, nausea, vision problems, enlargement of the ovaries and the development of ovarian cysts. Women on IVF programs are often receiving higher dosages than recommended by drug companies.[26]

There are a considerable number of studies indicating chromosomal problems with the eggs produced through this stimulation, and some studies indicate a structural similarity between clomiphene citrate and DES. A possible connection between the drug and both ovarian and breast cancer has been reported.[27] [28] The level of risk and danger associated with this drug does not justify its continued use on women both in IVF and in conventional infertility treatment.[29]

Considering the dangers to women and the expense involved, one Canadian clinic, the Queen Elizabeth Hospital in Montreal, shut down its IVF clinic in 1987. It had had no pregnancy since 1983 and no births. Dr Peter Cook, a former co-director of the clinic said that he and his colleagues had asked themselves 'Would I want my daughter or wife to undergo this procedure?' 'Given the reality, the answer was no,' he said.[30]

It is clear that IVF, while being considered by some researchers as a failed technology (because there is only a 4.8 per cent unproblematic live birth rate), represents an enormous cost to society and needs to be regulated.

Moreover, at each stage of the procedure, some women are dropped off the program—if, for example, their eggs cannot be collected or do not fertilise. An indication of the figures for this can be seen in the case of the Infertility Medical Centre at Epworth Hospital where the Monash team works. At this centre, 15 per cent of women are cancelled out at the egg collection stage and 35 per cent are cancelled at the embryo transfer stage.

Research scientists certainly want to remain a law unto themselves. They are so concerned about the possible creation of legislation in other states which might resemble that in Victoria that they have lobbied and used every means of persuasion to prevent this. These means include direct approaches to government committees, the use of old-boy networks, and the use of a professional lobbyist in Canberra.

The IVF lobby threatens that infertile couples will suffer, and that researchers will leave the country if there is legislation to restrict their activities. They will pick up their toys and find another sandpit. The Monash Medical Team has a history of this performance. It is often accompanied by stories of large amounts of money to be made overseas by doctors presently too patriotic to take up the offer. In 1985 Professor Carl Wood intimated that if IVF Australia was not allowed to proceed, the team would leave and had been offered 'two to three times what they earned in Melbourne'. In 1986 we read 'angry IVF doctors threaten to go abroad' after the Victorian Infertility Medical Procedures Act was passed. And in the science journal, *Nature*, in January 1987 we read that Dr Alan Trounson has 'issued an ultimatum that he and his team would go overseas within six months if they were not allowed to continue research'.

Doctors also promise that the medical profession will be self-regulating, that we can leave it to the professional bodies already established to take care of the ethics of our society. But their behaviour does not give us much faith in their ethics. We have already seen that experiments such as those using DES and concerning cervical cancer in New Zealand were not stopped by hospital ethics committees. And we have seen, in Victoria and Western Australia, doctors deliberately ignoring the advice of ethics committees constituted in order to convey the wishes of society with respect to these technologies.

In Victoria, scientists argued to change the law to allow embryo experimentation. During a significant and bloody battle, it was argued that they could not go ahead with micro-injection techniques because they needed to test whether the resulting embryo was healthy before implanting it into a woman. Yet even while discussions were still going on about changing the law, scientists went ahead with the micro-injection of women experimental subjects, not waiting for the law to be proclaimed.[31] Though its members constantly use their professional standing in order to convince us that they can regulate themselves, the medical profession shows itself to lack ethical credibility, sidestepping the law and the control of the community in this field. Where there is so much profit to be made, they cannot be the guardians of our ethical values.

Legislation is definitely needed in all of these spheres. The Victorian legislation has many faults, but so far Victoria is the only state which has had the courage to attempt to control the scientific research which is changing the nature of being human. What I have not covered in this paper are the many interconnected technologies related to IVF: embryo experimentation, sex predetermination, genetic manipulation and the development of the in vitro womb; the potential use of neomorts (someone newly dead) for both surrogacy and use as spare parts; and the increasing use of foetal tissue. Research in all these areas is ongoing and, unless the community takes control through legislation, it is medical research that will step into the breach to determine the nature of our society.

The final element in the social context of IVF is the issue of choice. Some women do claim the 'right' to use reproductive technology, regardless of the possible danger to their own bodies and the assault on their integrity. They also disregard the interrelationships between IVF and various other technologies such as genetic engineering, and the resulting implications that this has for our society.

But women's 'choices' are structured within a male-controlled political and social framework. Women do not as yet control abortion, contraception or the definitions of sexuality and relationships within that framework, and will not be in a position of control with respect to reproductive and genetic engineering. Even if that control were possible, the technologies themselves should not be allowed to continue because of the dangers involved for society as a whole and for women as a social group.

Abortion rights themselves are threatened by the new reproductive technologies. The medical profession currently colludes with women in ensuring abortion availability in most cases. But part of the rationale for this was to allow medical science to pursue prenatal screening techniques such as amniocentesis. There would be no point in developing these technologies if abortion were not available because the 'cure' for the 'disabilities' detected through these technologies was not available. Abortion was the sole solution and end result of the screening process. But once technology such as embryo biopsy and the screening of embryos *before* implantation becomes available, doctors will in all probability withdraw their support for abortion in favour of the screening of embryos and their elimination if 'unsatisfactory'.

Individual 'choice' as an argument in favour of reproductive technology fails to take into account the other element of the feminist value system—responsibility to women as a social group. There are times when the desires (not 'rights') of individual women have to be set aside because the fulfilment of those desires not only endangers individuals, but endangers the lives, integrity and survival of all women.

We must not delude ourselves into thinking that by using the word 'choice' we create it. I would argue that women are merely making a decision between two negative alternatives—and that is not a choice as feminism would define it. The decision between remaining childless and infertile in a world where women's worth is regarded only through motherhood, or undertaking a dangerous, expensive and failed technology, is not a choice that feminism would create. Only when women are materially, economically, politically, socially and ideologically equal to men can the experience of choice become a reality.

We must struggle to create real options for women in living their lives, including remaining childless and finding value in our lives without motherhood, and in creating a new concept of 'family' where women who choose not to have children, or women who cannot have them, can be included in permanent relationships with children and mothers, becoming part of the rearing of children in a new and less possessive way.

Reproductive technology does not take place outside of a social and political context. Practitioners and scientists running research programs in order to make profit are not best placed to make decisions about the future nature of our society.

Women are primarily involved here because it is women's bodies on whom the experimentation is taking place and it is women who will have to carry genetically manipulated embryos to term in order for science to determine whether their toying with the human building block has been effective. It is women who undergo the perilous procedures of IVF.

We must work to assist women to resist entering into these programs by looking at the underlying values of our society, which wrongly say that a woman is only whole if she is a mother. We need to resist the fragmentation and dismemberment of women's bodies which reproductive technology represents. We should abandon technologies like IVF which are dangerous, expensive and do not work. And we need to legislate to control medical research so that it is accountable to the society which it will either harm or assist into the future.

Notes

1 A version of this paper was delivered in Perth in January 1989, in debate with Dr John Yovich, at the University of Western Australia Summer School

2 Easlea, Brian *Science and Sexual Oppression: Patriarchy's Confrontation with Woman and Nature* London: Weidenfeld and Nicolson, 1981

3 Veitch, Andrew *The Guardian*

4 Scully, Diana *Men Who Control Women's Health* Boston: Houghton Mifflin, 1980; Direcks, Anita and Holmes, Helen Bequaert 'Miracle Drug, Miracle Baby' *New Scientist* 6 November 1986, 53–5; Driscol, Shirley G. and Taylor, Stephen H. 'Effects of Prenatal Maternal Estrogen on the Male Urogenital System' *Obstetrics and Gynaecology* 65, 5, 1980, 537–42; Corea, Gena *The Hidden Malpractice* New York: Harper and Row, 1985

5 Muasher, Suheil, Garcia, Jairo and Jones, Howard 'Experience with Diethylstilboestrol-Exposed Infertile Women in a Program of In Vitro Fertilisation' *Fertility and Sterility* 42, 1, 1984, 20–24

6 Coney, Sandra *The Unfortunate Experiment: The Full Story Behind the Inquiry Into Cervical Cancer Treatment* Ringwood, Vic: Penguin, 1988

7 Corea, Gena *Sortir La Maternité du Laboratoire* Quebec: Conseil Du Statut De Le Femme, 1988

8 'Low IVF Pregnancy Rate Tied to "Wayward Embryos" ' *Ob/Gyn News* 15 October 1986

9 Rowland, Robyn and Yovich, John *Public Debate University of Western Australia Summer School* 24 January 1989

10 'Coroner: "Omission" By Anaesthetist to IVF Death' *Geelong Advertiser* 29 November 1988; Trounson, Alan Debate on *'Tonight with Paul Murphy'* SBS Television, 6 June 1988

11 Fathalla, M. 'Incessant Ovulation; A Factor in Ovarian Neoplasia?' *The Lancet* 2, 163, 1971

12 Trounson, Alan *Report in Response to the Report of the Enquiry into Human Fertilisation and Embryology by the Medical Research Council, London, Passed on to the ASCHE* 1985, 6

13 McBain, John and Trounson, Alan 'Patient Management-Treatment Cycle' in Carl Wood and Alan Trounson (eds) *Clinical In Vitro Fertilisation* Berlin: Springer-Verlag, 1984, 54

14 Schumpeter, Peter, 'Why We are in Debt to Entrepreneurs' *The Age* 7 April 1986; Now In Vitro Gives Birth to Business Venture' *West Australian* 18 July 1985

15 Martin, Catherine 'A New and Fertile Field for Investment' *The Bulletin* 24 June 1986, Thorpe, Deryn 'IVF Enterprise Now Exported World Wide' *The Australian* 18 January 1988

16 ibid.

17 Blakeslee, Sandra 'Trying to Make Money Making Test Tube Babies' the *New York Times* 17 May 1987

18 Martin, Catherine, *op. cit.*

19 Cullen, Jenny 'Why we are losing IVF Researchers' *The Australian* 14 October 1986

20 'Land of the Raising Son' *Sunday Press* 12 February 1989

21 Klein, Renate *Infertility, Women Speak Out About Their Experiences of Reproductive Medicine* London: Pandora Press, 1989; Burton, Barbara 'Contentious Issues of Infertility Therapy—A Consumer's View', paper presented to the Australian Family Planning Association Annual Conference, March 1985; Crowe, Christine 'Women Want It: In Vitro Fertilisation and Women's Motivations for Participation' *Women's Studies International Forum* 1985, 457–552; Klein, Renate and Rowland, Robyn 'Women as Test-Sites for Fertility Drugs: Clomiphene Citrate and Hormonal Cocktails' *Reproductive and Genetic Engineering; Journal of International Feminist Analysis* 1, 3, 1988, 251–75

22 *In Vitro Fertilisation in Australia* Commonwealth Government Report, 1988

23 Bartels, Ditta 'High Failure Rates in In Vitro Fertilisation Treatments' *The Medical Journal of Australia* 16 November 1987, 474–5

24 *Finrrage Newsletter* May 1988, 5

25 *In Vitro Fertilisation in Australia, op. cit.*

26 Klein, *op. cit.* and Klein and Rowland, *op. cit.*

27 Carter, Marianne and Joyce, David N. 'Ovarian Carcinoma in Patient Hyperstimulated by Gonadotrophin Therapy for In Vitro Fertilisation: A Case Report' *Journal of In Vitro Fertilisation and Embryo Transfer* 4, 2, 1987, 126–8;

28 Bolton, P. M. 'Bilateral Breast Cancer Associated with Clomiphene' *The Lancet* 3 December 1977, 1176

29 Klein and Rowland, *op. cit.*

30 Pappert, Ann 'Success Rates Quoted by In Vitro Clinics Not What They Seem' *The Globe and Mail* 8 February 1988

31 Voumard, Sonya 'Suprise at Move to Apply IVF Technique' *The Age* 1988, 24

Index